Structural Competency in Mental Health and Medicine

Helena Hansen • Jonathan M. Metzl
Editors

Structural Competency in Mental Health and Medicine

A Case-Based Approach to Treating the Social Determinants of Health

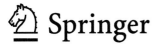 Springer

Editors
Helena Hansen
New York University
New York, NY
USA

Jonathan M. Metzl
Center for Medicine, Health, and Society
Vanderbilt University
Nashville, TN
USA

ISBN 978-3-030-10524-2   ISBN 978-3-030-10525-9   (eBook)
https://doi.org/10.1007/978-3-030-10525-9

Library of Congress Control Number: 2019935847

This Springer imprint is published by the registered company Springer Nature Switzerland AG
The registered company address is: Gewerbestrasse 11, 6330 Cham, Switzerland

Foreword: The Promise of Structural Competency

In 1966, Dr. Martin Luther King, Jr., singled out one form of inequality as especially egregious: "Of all the forms of inequality, injustice in health is the most shocking and inhuman."[1] Health disparities are not just a biological reality; they are a form of social inequality because they are structured according to unjust power arrangements. Numerous studies have established that the best predictor of health is an individual's position in the social order.[2] Poor health is a function of occupying a disadvantaged position in our society, while having better health is a benefit of being socially privileged. Similarly, people of color in the United States experience greater rates of morbidity and mortality than whites.[3] Dr. King's interpretation of health disparities as a key form of injustice also highlights how biological and cultural explanations for racial gaps in health help to support an unjust social order.

For centuries, dominant approaches to medicine and public health in the United States have woefully mistreated health inequities. Doctors and clinicians have not only ignored structural causes of health disparities; they have also helped to perpetuate unequal social structures. By attributing gaps in health to the innate or cultural traits of socially disadvantaged groups, medical professionals have obscured the very existence of political oppression. The racial concept of disease – that people of different races have different diseases and suffer from common diseases differently – has served since the slavery era to explain away the toll of oppression on African Americans and even to justify subordinating them for medical reasons. Dr. Samuel Cartwright, a well-known expert on "Negro medicine" before the Civil War, claimed that because black people had lower lung capacity than whites, forced labor

---

[1] *Dr. Martin Luther King on Health Care Injustice*, PHYSICIANS FOR A NAT'L HEALTH PROGRAM (Oct. 14, 2014), http://www.pnhp.org/news/2014/october/dr-martin-luther-king-on-health-care-injustice

[2] *See* DONALD A. BARR, HEALTH DISPARITIES IN THE UNITED STATES: SOCIAL CLASS, RACE, ETHNICITY, AND HEALTH (2008); Nancy E. Adler & David H. Rehkopf, *U.S. Disparities in Health: Descriptions, Causes, and Mechanisms*, 29 ANN. REV. PUB. HEALTH 235 (2008).

[3] *See* NAT'L CTR. FOR HEALTH STATISTICS, CTR. FOR DISEASE CONTROL AND PREVENTION, HEALTH, UNITED STATES 2015: WITH SPECIAL FEATURE ON RACIAL & ETHNIC HEALTH DISPARITIES 37–38, 100–01 (May 2016), http://www.cdc.gov/nchs/data/hus/hus15.pdf; Robert S. Levine, James E. Foster & Robert E. Fullilove, *Black-White Inequalities in Mortality and Life Expectancy, 1933–1999: Implications for Health People 2010*, 116 PUB. HEALTH REP. 474, 480 (2001); David R. Williams, *Miles To Go Before We Sleep: Racial Inequities in Health*, 53 J. HEALTH & SOC. BEHAV. 279, 280 (2012).

was good for them.[4] Locating blacks' subordinated status in biological susceptibility later legitimized the white supremacist regime inherited from slavery.

The explanation for health disparities as caused by innate distinctions in disease diverts attention and resources from ending health disparities' structural causes and perpetuates the false belief that social inequality stems from biological differences. Using biological terms to define social inequities makes them seem natural – the result of inherent group differences that can't be changed instead of unjust societal structures that must be dismantled. Attributing health disparities to cultural differences in health behaviors makes them seem the fault of the very groups who face the greatest structural barriers to good health and well being. These ways of thinking serve as a powerful barrier to support for structural changes needed to create a more equal society in which everyone would be healthier.

We have long known that health inequities are caused by the structural determinants of health. A growing field of empirical research demonstrates that racism negatively affects the health of African Americans through a variety of pathways.[5] Scientists are now uncovering the biological pathways that translate inequities in wealth, employment, health care, housing, incarceration, and education, along with experiences of stigma and discrimination, into disparate health outcomes. Institutionalized racism in these systems restricts access to resources required for health and well being. Numerous studies have identified racially segregated housing as a key contributor to health disparities because it concentrates poverty and minimizes resources needed for good health in predominantly black neighborhoods.[6] As a group of health researchers recently summarized, racial residential segregation harms health through multiple pathways, including "the high concentration of dilapidated housing in neighbourhoods that people of color reside in, the substandard quality of the social and built environment, exposure to pollutants and toxins, limited opportunities for high-quality education and decent employment, and restricted access to health care."[7] In addition, the psychosocial stressors related to living in a high-poverty neighborhood are intensified by stress stemming from racial discrimination in health care, schools, employment, foster care, prisons, and policing that prevails in these same areas.[8] By geographically concentrating racism and

---

[4] LUNDY BRAUN, BREATHING RACE INTO THE MACHINE: THE SURPRISING CAREER OF THE SPIROMETER FROM PLANTATION TO GENETICS 28 (2014).

[5] *See*, e.g., Elizabeth Brondolo, Linda C. Gallo & Hector F. Myers, *Race, Racism and Health: Disparities, Mechanisms, and Interventions*, 32 J. BEHAV. MED. 1 (2009); David R. Williams & Selina A. Mohammed, *Racism and Health I: Pathways and Scientific Evidence*, 57 AM. BEHAV. SCI. 1152 (2013); Zinzi D. Bailey et al., *Structural Racism and Health Inequities in the USA: Evidence and Interventions*, 389 THE LANCET 1453, 1456–58 (2017).

[6] *See* David R. Williams & Chiquita Collins, *Racial Residential Segregation: A Fundamental Cause of Racial Disparities in Health*, 116 PUB. HEALTH REP. 404, 410–11 (2001); Williams & Muhammed, at 1158–59.

[7] Bailey et al., at 1456; Williams & Muhammed, at 1159.

[8] *See* Camara Jules P. Harrell et al., *Multiple Pathways Linking Racism to Health Outcomes*, 8 DU BOIS REV. 143, 153 (2011); Nancy Krieger, *Discrimination and Health Inequities*, 44 INT'L J. HEALTH SERVS. 643, 652–54 (2014); Williams & Mohammed, at 1163–64.

poverty, residential segregation creates neighborhood environments for black residents that are extraordinarily destructive to their health.

Yet the biological and cultural accounts of racial and other health disparities continue to shape medical ideas and practices today.[9] Medical education in the United States typically perpetuates biological concepts of race, the racial concept of disease, and stereotypes about racial differences that contribute to inferior treatment of black patients. Treating patients by race is still a foundation of medical education: students are routinely taught to identify a patient's race and to use it as a proxy for more important clinical factors. At the same time, public health and biomedical researchers increasingly focus on genetic differences to explain health disparities. Rather than grapple with racist ideas embedded in the curriculum, medical schools have sought to address physician bias by requiring students, interns, and residents to be trained in "cultural competency" to better understand patient lifestyles and attitudes.[10] Cultural competency training is supposed to help health care professionals communicate with patients of differing ethnic backgrounds and understand the cultural factors that influence patients' health behaviors.

Neither of these approaches – the biological or the cultural – attends to the structural forces that actually drive health disparities and have a tremendous impact on people's well being. Health inequities should be addressed by training health professionals to be more *structurally* competent.[11] As Jonathan M. Metzl and I wrote elsewhere, "locating medical approaches to racial diversity solely in the bodies, backgrounds, or attitudes of patients and doctors, therefore, leaves practitioners unprepared to address the biological, socioeconomic, and racial impacts of upstream decisions on structural factors such as expanding health and wealth disparities."[12] The growing movement for "structural competency" radically departs from these biological and cultural approaches by contending that "many health-related factors previously attributed to culture or ethnicity also represent the downstream consequences of decisions about larger structural contexts, including health care and food delivery systems, zoning laws, local politics, urban and rural infrastructures, structural racisms, or even the very definitions of illness and health."[13] Health care providers need to be more competent at recognizing and addressing these upstream structural factors that determine patients' health and create health inequities.

---

[9] JOHN HOBERMAN, BLACK AND BLUE: THE ORIGINS AND CONSEQUENCES OF MEDICAL RACISM 32–37 (2012); BRAUN, at 164; DOROTHY ROBERTS, FATAL INVENTION: HOW SCIENCE, POLITICS, AND BIG BUSINESS RE-CREATE RACE IN THE TWENTY-FIRST CENTURY 57–80, 104–122 (2012).

[10] Sunil Kripalani et al., *A Prescription for Cultural Competence in Medical Education*, 21 J. GEN. INTERNAL MED. 1116 (2006).

[11] Jonathan Metzl & Helena Hansen, Structural competency: theorizing a new medical engagement with stigma and inequality. 103 *Soc Sci Med.* 126 (2014).

[12] Jonathan M. Metzl & Dorothy E. Roberts, *Structural Competency Meets Structural Racism: Race, Politics, and the Structure of Medical Knowledge*, 9 AM. MED. ASS'N. J. OF ETHICS 674 (2014), https://journalofethics.ama-assn.org/article/structural-competency-meets-structural-racism-race-politics-and-structure-medical-knowledge

[13] Metzl & Roberts, 674.

Structural competency is revolutionary. It not only addresses the negative impact of structural inequalities on health but forges a path to undo medicine's support for an unjust social order. It reverses the paradigm of biological and cultural excuses for maintaining the unequal social structure to reveal the importance of dismantling the unequal social structure in order to improve health. Structural competency radically rejects the ideology that attributes social injustice to biological differences and replaces it with an ideology that takes account of the biological harms caused by social injustice. It radically rejects the exclusive focus on individual responsibility for one's own health outcomes and replaces it with public responsibility for creating the conditions needed for health and well being. And it radically transforms the relationship between medical professionals and the communities they serve from one of arrogant authority over patients to recognizing the competencies and expertise patients and their communities offer. It requires, as well, alliances with other disciplines and movements for social, economic, and environmental justice to have the capacity to achieve structural change. Thus, structural competency is more than a critique of existing approaches to medicine; it is also a positive model for systemic intervention to improve health and create a more equal society.

This path breaking *Structural Competency Casebook* is critical to achieving structural competency's radical promise. By providing case studies where structural competency has operated successfully, Helena Hansen, Jonathan M. Metzl, and the contributing authors show us not only why we need to change medical education and practice but how to do it. It can be dispiriting to tell doctors, nurses, clinicians, and students only about the harms medicine has inflicted; they also need to know what they can do to change medical practice and work toward social transformations. These cases give us a blueprint for putting structural competency into practice and inspiration to envision the difference it can make for a better world.

Dorothy E. Roberts
George A. Weiss University Professor of Law & Sociology
University of Pennsylvania
Philadelphia, PA, USA

Acknowledgements

In addition to the authors contributing to this volume, we wish to thank Laura G. Duncan, Sewitt Bereket, Matthew Schneider, Sonia Mendoza, Meagan Artus, Philip Pettis, and Mia Keeys for their invaluable organization of the meetings and communication leading up to this book.

We also wish to thank Sayantani Dasgupta, Sue Estroff, Bruce Link, Jo Phelan, Nancy Scheper-Hughes, Kamini Doobay, Kim Hopper, Jennifer Van Tiem, James Quesada, Rayna Rapp, Emily Martin, Alondra Nelson, Michael Ralph, Dalton Conley, Dolores Malaspina, Kathryn Church, Irene Matheiu, Nancy Angoff, Nichole Roxas, Gary Belkin, Marc Gourevitch, Bradley Lewis, Neely Myers, Mehret Mandefro, Mary Louise Pratt, Sharon Kaufman, Derek Griffith, Kim Sue, Sally Lehrman, Vincanne Adams, Babak Tofighi, Philip Alberti, Denise Herd, Dorothy Porter, Laurence J. Kirmayer, Rachel Kronick, Cécile Rousseau, Cameron Donald, Kristen Eckstrand, Diane Dao, Adeline Goss, Andrew Hoekzema, Lauren Kelly, Alexander Logan, Sanjiv Mehta, Utpal Sandesara, Michelle R. Munyikwa, Horace M. DeLisser, Stef Bertozzi, Rupa Marya, Shirley Strong, John Balmes, Michel Cantal-Dupart, Adam Reich, Danielle Celermajer, Kenneth Anderson, Robert Haemmig, Robert Heimer, Dan Small, Alex Walley, Evan Wood, and Ingrid van Beek for their intellectual engagement with the authors and editors of this book during its development.

The financial and in-kind support of the NYU Department of Psychiatry, Department of Anthropology, Department of Social and Cultural Analysis, as well as the New York State Office of Mental Health at the Nathan Kline Institute for Psychiatric Research, the Vanderbilt Center for Medicine, Health, and Society, and the Kaiser Permanente Foundation were indispensible for completing this book.

Contents

Part II   Structural Competency in Non-health Sector Collaborations

Part III   Structural Competency in Community Engagement

Part IV   Structural Competency in Policy Advocacy

About the Authors

Helena Hansen MD, Ph.D., is Associate Professor in the Departments of Anthropology and Psychiatry at NYU. She has published widely in clinical and social science journals on faith healing of addiction in Puerto Rico, psychiatric disability under U.S. welfare reform, addiction pharmaceuticals and race, ethnic marketing of pharmaceuticals, and structural competency. Her book *Addicted to Christ: Remaking Men in Puerto Rican Pentecostal Drug Ministries* was published by UC Press in 2018. Her current ethnographic study of the introduction of new addiction pharmaceuticals examines the social and political implications of clinicians' efforts to establish addiction as a biomedical, rather than moral or social condition, as well as the ways that neurochemical treatments reinscribe hierarchies of ethnicity and race, has led to a second book project on how the current opioid crisis became "white," as well as a feature length documentary, *Managing the Fix*. She has received major funding from NIDA, the Mellon Foundation, and the Robert Wood Johnson Foundation. She is the recipient of the Kaiser Permanente Burche Minority Leadership Award, the Golden Dozen Teaching Award, and the American Association of Directors of Psychiatry Residency Training Model Curriculum Award.

Jonathan M. Metzl MD, Ph.D., (@jonathanmetzl) is the Frederick B. Rentschler II Professor of Sociology and Psychiatry, and the Director of the Center for Medicine, Health, and Society, at Vanderbilt University in Nashville, Tennessee. He received his MD from the University of Missouri, MA in humanities/poetics and Psychiatric internship/residency from Stanford University, and PhD in American Culture from University of Michigan, A 2008 Guggenheim fellow, Professor Metzl has written extensively for medical, psychiatric, and popular publications. His books include *Dying of Whiteness, The Protest Psychosis, Prozac on the Couch,* and *Against Health: How Health Became the New Morality.*

Contributors

Andrew F. Beck, MD, MPH Divisions of General & Community Pediatrics and Hospital Medicine, Cincinnati Children's Hospital Medical Center, Cincinnati, OH, USA

Department of Pediatrics, University of Cincinnati College of Medicine, Cincinnati, OH, USA

Gary Belkin, MD, MPH, PhD NYC Department of Health and Mental Hygiene, New York City, NY, USA

Department of Psychiatry, New York University School of Medicine, New York City, NY, USA

Philippe Bourgois, PhD Semel Institute of Neuroscience, Department Psychiatry and Biobehavioral Sciences, David Geffen School of Medicine, University of California, Los Angeles, Los Angeles, CA, USA

Joel T. Braslow, MD, PhD UCLA David Geffen School of Medicine, University of California, Los Angeles, Los Angeles, CA, USA

Billy Bromage, MSW Department of Psychiatry, Yale School of Medicine, New Haven, CT, USA

Gregory Chin Department of Neurological Surgery, University of California, San Francisco, San Francisco, CA, USA

Edgar Rivera Colón, PhD Narrative Medicine Program, Columbia University, New York, NY, USA

Saint Peter's University, The Jesuit University of New Jersey, Jersey City, NJ, USA

Jeffrey Coots, JD, MPH Department of Criminal Justice, John Jay College of Criminal Justice, City University of New York, New York City, NY, USA

Mallory Curran, JD Mallory Curran Consulting, Brooklyn, NY, USA

Jorge De Avila University of Chicago Pritzker School of Medicine, Chicago, IL, USA

Cameron Donald, MS University of California, San Francisco, San Francisco, CA, USA

Ernest Drucker, PhD New York University, College of Global Public Health, New York City, NY, USA

Montefiore Medical Center/Albert Einstein College of Medicine, New York City, NY, USA

Sam Dubal, MD, PhD Department of Medical Anthropology, University of California, Berkeley, Berkeley, CA, USA

University of California, San Francisco, San Francisco, CA, USA

Laura G. Duncan Medical Scientist Training Program, Department of Anthropology, History and Social Medicine, University of California, San Francisco, San Francisco, CA, USA

Pyser S. Edelsack, MSW Sophie Davis School of Biomedical Education, City University of New York Medical School, New York, NY, USA

John A. Encandela, PhD Teaching and Learning Center, Yale School of Medicine, New Haven, CT, USA

Fabián Fernández, MPH University of California, San Francisco, San Francisco, CA, USA

Mindy Thompson Fullilove, MD The New School, New York, NY, USA

Robert E. Fullilove III, EdD Mailman School of Public Health, Columbia University, New York, NY, USA

Jack Geiger, MD, MSciHyg Department of Community Health and Social Medicine, Sophie Davis School of Biomedical Education, City University of New York Medical School, New York, NY, USA

Jeremy A. Greene, MD, PhD Department of the History of Medicine, Center for Medical Humanities and Social Medicine, Johns Hopkins University School of Medicine, Baltimore, MD, USA

Jodi Halpern, MD, PhD UC Berkeley-UCSF Joint Medical Program, Berkeley, CA, USA

Helena Hansen, MD, PhD New York University, New York City, NY, USA

Michael Harvey, DrPH San Jose State University, San Jose, CA, USA

Adrienne W. Henize, JD Division of General and Community Pediatrics, Cincinnati Children's Hospital Medical Center, Cincinnati, OH, USA

Seth M. Holmes, MD, PhD Division of Society and Environment, Joint Program in Medical Anthropology, Berkeley Center for Social Medicine, University of California, Berkeley, Berkeley, CA, USA

Elaine Hsiang, BA University of California, San Francisco, San Francisco, CA, USA

Nadia Islam, PhD Department of Population Health, NYU School of Medicine, New York, NY, USA

Alethia Jones, PhD Open Society Foundations Fellowships Program, New York, NY, USA

Molly Rose Kaufman, MS University of Orange, Orange, NJ, USA

Talha Khan Sophie Davis School of Biomedical Education, City University of New York Medical School, New York, NY, USA

Melissa D. Klein, MD, MEd Division of General and Community Pediatrics, Cincinnati Children's Hospital Medical Center, Cincinnati, OH, USA

Kelly Ray Knight, PhD Department of Anthropology, History and Social Medicine, University of California, San Francisco, San Francisco, CA, USA

Elaine Lemay Samuel Merritt University, Oakland, CA, USA

Brett Lewis Oregon Health Sciences University, Portland, OR, USA

Walter S. Mathis, MD Department of Psychiatry, Yale School of Medicine, New Haven, CT, USA

Jenifer Matthews, MD Department of Adolescent Medicine, University of California San Francisco Benioff Children's Hospital Oakland, Oakland, CA, USA

Aimee Medeiros, PhD Department of Anthropology, History and Social Medicine, University of California, San Francisco, San Francisco, CA, USA

Omar Mesina, BA University of California, San Francisco, San Francisco, CA, USA

Jonathan M. Metzl, MD, PhD Center for Medicine, Health, and Society, Vanderbilt University, Nashville, TN, USA

Michael J. Montoya, PhD Anthropology & Chicanx/Latinx Studies, School of Social Sciences, Program in Medical Education for the Latino Community, School of Medicine, Public Health & Nursing Science, College of Health Sciences, University of California, Irvine, Irvine, CA, USA

Graham Mooney, PhD Institute of the History of Medicine, Center for Medical Humanities and Social Medicine, Johns Hopkins University School of Medicine, Department of Epidemiology, Baltimore, MD, USA

Joshua Neff, MS UC Berkeley-UCSF Joint Medical Program, Berkeley, CA, USA

Nick Nelson, MBBS Internal Medicine Residency Program, Highland Hospital, Oakland, CA, USA

University of California, San Francisco, San Francisco, CA, USA

Julie Netherland, PhD Drug Policy Alliance, New York City, NY, USA

Donita S. Parrish, JD Legal Aid Society of Greater Cincinnati, Cincinnati, OH, USA

Parth Patel Mount Sinai Medical Center, Miami Beach, FL, USA

Edward G. Paul, MD Department of Family Medicine, St. Joseph's Hospital & Medical Center/Dignity Health, Phoenix, AZ, USA

Philip J. Pettis, LMSW Department of Sociology, Vanderbilt University, Nashville, TN, USA

JuLeigh Petty, PhD Center for Medicine, Health, and Society, Vanderbilt University, Nashville, TN, USA

Lourdes Rodriguez, DrPH Center for Place-Based Initiatives, Dell Medical School, Austin, TX, USA

University of Austin, Texas, Austin, TX, USA

Robert M. Rohrbaugh, MD Department of Psychiatry, Office of International Medical Student Education, Yale School of Medicine, New Haven, CT, USA

Sarah Rosenwohl-Mack, MPH University of California, San Francisco, San Francisco, CA, USA

Shannon Satterwhite Medical Scientist Training Program, Department of Anthropology, History and Social Medicine, University of California, San Francisco, San Francisco, CA, USA

Jack Saul, PhD International Trauma Studies Program, New York City, NY, USA

Virginia T. Spell, BA Urban League of Southern Connecticut, Stamford, CT, USA

Shirley Strong, MEd Samuel Merritt University, Oakland, CA, USA

Carolyn Sufrin, MD, PhD Department of Gynecology and Obstetrics, Center for Medical Humanities and Social Medicine, Johns Hopkins School of Medicine, Baltimore, MD, USA

Department of Health, Behavior, and Society, Johns Hopkins Bloomberg School of Public Health, Baltimore, MD, USA

Judith Sugarman Center for Urban and Community Services, New York, NY, USA

Selena Suhail-Sindhu, MPH New York University, New York City, NY, USA

MD Taher, MPH Department of Population Health, NYU School of Medicine, New York, NY, USA

Ariana Thompson-Lastad, PhD Osher Center for Integrative Medicine, University of California, San Francisco, San Francisco, CA, USA

Elizabeth Tobin-Tyler, JD, MA Department of Family Medicine, Warren Alpert Medical School of Brown University, Providence, RI, USA

Department of Health Services, Policy and Practice, Brown University School of Public Health, Providence, RI, USA

Chau Trinh-Shevrin, DrPH Department of Population Health, NYU School of Medicine, New York, NY, USA

Lily Walkover, PhD Global Health, Drexel University, Philadelphia, PA, USA

Bridgett Williamson Department of Psychiatry, Yale School of Medicine, New Haven, CT, USA

Introduction

This book represents one answer to a question that contributors received from colleagues, namely: "I like the idea of structural competency – the idea that as clinicians we should work to change the structural causes of unequal health among our patients – but how do you actually put it into practice?" In response, this book explores how theoretical concepts central to structural competency work in the real worlds of clinical practice and medical education, and imparts lessons for adapting key lessons into new locales.

To be clear, this is *not* a "how to" manual, because a manual would be too formulaic and mechanical for an undertaking that requires creativity and flexibility. Rather, this book presents narratives of successful interventions in clinical training and practice that highlight what is possible to do as clinicians, students, and health workers, in collaboration with others who have complementary expertise. By definition, structural competency aims to draw on local strengths and resources for the difficult work of changing social structures (such as improving neighborhood quality through community organizations, or integrating health-related interventions into non-health sector agencies like housing, education and law enforcement, or collaborating with policy makers). The strategies that are successful in New York cannot simply be grafted on to San Francisco, Philadelphia, Nashville, or rural Wisconsin.

As the chapters in this book detail, *structural competency* attempts to bridge the gap between individual and institutional drivers of inequality, or between what racism and other forms of discrimination in medicine are and what they do. Whereas earlier models such as cultural competency focused mainly on identifying clinician bias and improving communication at moments of clinical encounter, structural competency emphasizes diagnostic recognition of the economic and political conditions that produce health inequalities in the first place. Structural competency also addresses the clinical effects of structural stigma and racism. As described in the 2014 publication that first theorized structural competency, "if stigmas are not primarily produced in individual encounters but are enacted there due to structural causes, it then follows that clinical training must shift its gaze from an exclusive focus on the individual encounter to include the organization of institutions and policies, as well as of neighborhoods and cities, if clinicians are to impact stigma-related health inequalities" [1].

The notion that health inequalities reflect social inequalities that are prefigured by public policies, economic structures, governmental and non-governmental agencies as well as neighborhood living conditions is not new. As physician Rudolf Virchow, a founder of modern pathology as well as public health research, said in 1848: "Medicine is a social science, and politics is nothing else but medicine on a large scale" [2]. However structural competency draws on the contemporary cachet of "competencies" in clinical education (as of this writing, the Association of American Medical Colleges promotes the training and measurement of medical students in 15 core competencies) [3] in order to hold clinicians accountable for learning not only about molecular, cellular, and organ structures that determine health, but also for learning about social institutional structures that are among the strongest drivers of their patients' health outcomes and about how to intervene on those institutions to improve health. The Afro-Caribbean physician and social theorist Frantz Fanon wrote in 1967, "What matters is not to know the world but to change it" [4]. In this spirit, the contributors to this book have come together under the umbrella of structural competency to describe their interventions to reduce health inequalities, but in their every day practice they use a range of other terms, ranging from social medicine, social determinants of health, upstream intervention, cultural humility, health justice, and anti-racism to health equity.

And how did the alliance of clinicians and advocates, materialized in this book, come about?

It was 2011. The editors of this book, Helena Hansen and Jonathan M. Metzl, had met at a national conference for MD-PhDs in the social sciences and humanities, on a panel which analyzed clinical case descriptions in terms of structural violence and institutional discrimination. Helena Hansen was a psychiatrist and anthropologist researching the structural drivers of race in drug policy, in particular of the "whiteness" of the US opioid crisis: the concerted action of pharmaceutical marketing, deregulation based on the idea whites were at lower risk for addiction than blacks and Latinos, as well as implicit racial imagery underlying neuroscience and biotech development based on an imagined middle class white narcotic consumer base [5, 6]. She had come of age when AIDS activism was peaking, and had seen first-hand how the sit-ins and "die-ins" of HIV positive people and politically active health workers had achieved historic changes in health practices and policies, fostering peer-led safer sex and harm reduction initiatives, requiring participation of HIV positive people on scientific review bodies and in the conduct of clinical trials. Years later, when she was asked to develop the curriculum in her psychiatry residency, she inverted what had been a cultural competency course into a course on the "culture of psychiatry and biomedicine" – the history, politics, and economics of clinical practice. Rather than asking residents to analyze the cultural beliefs and behaviors of their patients, the course asked residents to consider how they could intervene on the structural drivers of health inequalities, including the institutions of biomedicine themselves.

Jonathan M. Metzl had just published the book *The Protest Psychosis: How Schizophrenia Became a Black Disease* [7]; in it he suggested that cultural competency training would not change the overdiagnosis of schizophrenia in Black men. Based on historical research on the evolution of the diagnosis of paranoid schizophrenia in response to angry Black men who surfaced in emergency rooms in the wake of 1960s of civil rights protests, Jonathan coined the term that frames this book, proposing that psychiatrists receive training in *structural competency* – the ways that diagnostic systems themselves reflect racially divergent patterns of pathologization, hospitalization, and resulting life chances. Looking closely at the ways that clinicians had traditionally learned to understand race and racism, he argued that healthcare providers and students needed to better recognize how institutions, markets, or healthcare delivery systems shape symptom presentations and to mobilize for correction of health and wealth inequalities in society.

Over lunch in Manhattan's Little India, the editors of this book discussed how to make "structural competency" into a "thing." Thinking of their attempts as physician-social scientists to bring social theories of institutions and ideologies that shape health outcomes into clinical training, and of their clinical colleagues' demand for practical intervention, not just concepts, they sketched a framework for clinical practice that targeted the social determinants of health on the back of a napkin.

They drew on the literature of critical race studies, anthropology, sociology, gender studies, economics, urban planning, and public health, to outline a series of benchmark skills to recognize and intervention on structural factors as they arise in clinical settings, including:

- *Recognizing the structures that shape clinical interactions:* Rather than interpreting patient presentations solely in terms of patients' beliefs and behaviors, clinicians also examine the social conditions and institutional policies that may have contributed to patient presentations.
- *Rearticulating "cultural" formulations in structural terms:* Clinicians develop diagnoses and treatment plans that account for neighborhood and institutional factors.
- *Observing and enacting structural interventions:* Practitioners work on community–, service agency–, or policy advocacy–based projects that address the systemic needs of their patient populations.
- *Developing structural humility:* Practitioners collaborate across disciplines and with community members, bearing in mind that systemic change often progresses slowly and requires long-term investment.

In the months and years that followed, the editors discovered a national network of colleagues in medical schools and clinics across the country who had long been working in a parallel process to inject social and structural determinants of health into clinical training and practice. Centers of activity had developed under the leadership of committed and insightful clinicians, social scientists, and community activists in places as far flung as Chapel Hill North Carolina, University of Chicago, Yale/New Haven, UCLA, Philadelphia, Boston, San Francisco, and Oregon. This expanding network started a dialog through national conferences (four of them on the theme of structural competency between 2012 and 2017), special journal issues (three of them on structural competency from 2016 to 2018 [9–11]), and a number of webinars and podcasts including those produced by the American Medical Student's Association and the New York State Department of Health.

Along the way, colleagues who had been active in the social medicine movements of the 1960s pointed out that structural competency was a reinvention of social medicine approaches that dated to before the industrial revolution. As H. Jack Geiger, renown 1960s social medicine physician and founder of the Community Health Center system that still brings federally funded healthcare to low-income areas across the country, reminded readers in a commentary that he wrote for an issue of *Academic Medicine* on structural competency that

> in 1790, Johann Peter Frank, the Austrian dean of an Italian Medical School, delivered a commencement address to newly credentialed young physicians called 'The People's Misery: Mother of All Diseases.' The economic, environmental, social and occupational conditions of the peasantry should be changed, and that effort should be part of a physician's work…[a century] later John Simon, the first health officer of London, wrote of the urban working class, 'living in some lightless feverbin, breathing from the cesspools and the sewer' and able to afford only stale bread and diluted milk for his children. His first official report called for parliament to act to change such conditions and provide financial and other support [8].

Yet, it is not obvious in this contemporary era how social medicine can be practiced. At each structural competency conference, and in response to each structural competency journal article and webinar, participants and readers asked what does structural competency training and structurally competent clinical practice actually look like in other settings? Which concrete interventions can I adapt to my own medical school, or practice, or neighborhood?

This book presents cases of structural competency interventions from members of our national network and places them into one of four levels of structural intervention. The first part, Structural Competency in Classrooms and Clinics, focuses on clinical education within the classroom. Cases in this part describe innovative work with a range of trainees, from premedical students enrolled in a new pre-health college major that centers on structural competency with grounding in scholarship from the medical social sciences and humanities (Metz et al., this volume, chapter "Teaching and Testing Structural Competency in Pre-health Undergraduate Classrooms"); to psychiatry residents and MD-PhD students in the social sciences and humanities (Braslow and Bourgois, this volume, chapter "Teaching Social Medicine as Applied Sociomedical Practice"); and to a collective of community activists, medical residents, and medical students that bring structural competency courses to a range of community settings and applications (Neff et al., this volume, chapter "The Structural Competency Working Group: Lessons from Iterative, Interdisciplinary Development of a Structural Competency Training Module"). Contributors to this part also describe reworking the contours of the classroom and training programs themselves; Greene et al. bring medical students out of the classroom and into the streets of Baltimore in order to witness firsthand the structures of neighborhood inequality that manifest in "hot spots" of poor health on geocoded health maps, while Knight et al. describe exchanges between medical student activists in White Coats for Black Lives and their medical school faculty members to retool the undergraduate curriculum to take up racism and social inequality as core topics. Colon tutors medical students in health and civil rights activism using history and literature, and Geiger et al. describe the redesign of an entire medical school around social justice, in the form of Sophie Davis School of Biomedical Education, a 7-year combined BA-MD program started by the City University of

New York over 40 years ago to recruit promising high school students of color from medically underserved communities into medicine, and which starts medical training by having students conduct community health assessments to identify social patterning of disease in their own neighborhoods.

The second part, Structural Competency in Non-Health Sector Collaborations, calls attention to the potential for clinical practitioners to align with urban planners, churches, youth and community centers, as well as lawyers within medical-legal partnerships. Fullilove et al. (this volume, chapter "Urbanism Is a Participatory Sport: Reflections on Teaching About Cities in a School of Public Health") show how public health practitioners can work with urban planners and architects to reduce race and class segregation in cities that is a major driver of health inequalities. Saul (this volume, chapter "Promoting Collective Recovery in an Immigrant/Refugee Community Following Massive Trauma") details the evolution of health interventions for a traumatized community of refugees from the Liberian War that ultimately took the form of a community center offering youth services and cultural arts. Beck et al. (this volume, chapter "Is Poverty Making Me Sick? An Example of the Impact of Medical-Legal Partnership on Keeping Children Healthy") highlight medical-legal partnerships as potent agents for individual and collective health justice, to challenge neglect and abuses by institutions, ranging from housing agencies to schools, that foster health inequalities. Collectively these cases help readers to redraw the boundaries of healthcare to encompass professional disciplines and sectors that are not traditionally included in health interventions.

The third part, Structural Competency in Community Engagement, takes this logic of expansion of healthcare beyond clinic walls a step further. It highlights the efforts of clinical faculty, trainees, and researchers to engage community organizations in providing comprehensive care which links patients with resources and support in their neighborhoods. Montoya (this volume, chapter "Relational Politics of Clinical Care: Lessons from the University of California PRIME-LC Program"), in developing a state-funded training program designed to improve health outcomes in Latinx communities in Southern California, highlights not only medical student participation in community organizing events, but also the skill of "accompaniment" – deep listening and presence by clinicians and researchers who ally themselves with community members' work toward self-determination. Rohrbaugh et al. (this volume, chapter "Allying with Our Neighbors to Teach Structural Competence: The Yale Department of Psychiatry Structural Competency Community Initiative (YSCCI)") provide experiential learning in which they have psychiatry residents not only to join local community members with lived experience of psychiatric treatment on a tour of the low-income neighborhoods from which many of their patients come, but also have residents to take public transportation to those neighborhoods, and to find a healthy lunch there for $2, the amount usually allotted to patients receiving public benefits. Chau et al. (this volume, chapter "Community Health Workers as Accelerators of Community Engagement and Structural Competency in Health") describe the integration of community health workers into blood glucose control interventions in South Asian communities with epidemic rates of diabetes, and Sindhu et al. describe a psychiatry residency training initiative that pairs residents with mental health peers specialists – people with lived experience with psychiatric treatment who work to support others who are psychiatrically diagnosed – to identify and visit community resources and to use what they learn to construct an interactive, online community resource map for use in patient care.

Finally, Structural Competency in Policy Advocacy, the fourth part of this book, examines the role of clinical practitioners and health workers in policy advocacy. Coots et al. (this volume, chapter "From Punishment to Public Health: Interdisciplinary Dialogues and Cross-Sector Policy Innovations") describe an organization made up of mental health practitioners, public health researchers, and disenchanted criminal justice administrators that works to divert people with serious psychiatric diagnoses from the carceral system toward mental healthcare. Their efforts have ranged from changing policing practices to provide mental health assessments prior to arrest, to lobbying the state legislature for changes in drug laws that reduce the incarceration of people with mental health and substance use disorders. In this vein, Netherland (this volume, chapter "Physicians as Policy Advocates: from the Clinic to the State House") documents the training provided by the Drug Policy Alliance for clinical practitioners to testify for lawmakers and to use their influence as health professionals to privilege health outcomes in policy reform. Jones (this volume, chapter "Agents of Change: How Allied Health Care Workers Transform Inequalities in the Healthcare Industry") focuses the lens of policy and health onto the healthcare industry itself, highlighting the historical and contemporary role of healthcare worker's unions in achieving structural changes such as livable wages and benefits that narrow inequalities within hospitals and clinics while providing a model for collective action to improve the health and well-being of workers in other industries.

At the end of this book, a bibliography and set of syllabi from cases of classroom interventions provide readers with practical resources for use in their own structural competency interventions.

This book represents one step toward a needed paradigm shift in clinical training and practice – a shift that emphasizes connections between clinics and communities, highlights the clinical effects of racism in addition to the health implications of race, and suggests how health "disparities" reflect dominant ideologies and practices in addition to minority ones. Many of the cases described were initiated and/or meaningfully developed by students and residents who were still in training, and by care providers from patient populations themselves, including mental health peers and community health workers, which is a promising sign for the future of structural competency. Only the energies and insights of the future generations of socially aware clinical practitioners, peer support providers, and community organizers will end social inequalities and institutional racism as primary determinants of health.

Helena Hansen
New York University, New York, NY, USA

Jonathan M. Metzl
Center for Medicine, Health, and Society
Vanderbilt University
Nashville, TN, USA

References

1. Metzl JM, Hansen H. Structural competency: theorizing a new medical engagement with stigma and inequality. Soc Sci Med 2014;103:126–33.
2. Mackenbach JP. Politics is nothing but medicine at a larger scale: reflections on public health's biggest idea. J Epidemiol Community Health 2009;63(3):181–4.
3. AAMC: Core Competencies for Entering Medical Students. 2018. https://www.aamc.org/admissions/dataandresearch/477182/corecompetencies.html.
4. Fanon F. Black skin, white masks. London: Paladin; 1970.
5. Netherland J, Hansen H. White opioids: pharmaceutical race and the war on drugs that wasn't. BioSocieties 2017;12(2):217–38.
6. Hansen H, Netherland J. Is the prescription opioid epidemic a white problem? Am J Public Health 2016 106(12):2127.
7. Metzl JM. The protest psychosis: how schizophrenia became a black disease. Boston: Beacon Press; 2010.
8. Geiger HJ. The political future of social medicine: reflections on physicians as activists. Acad Med 2017;92(3):282–4.
9. Metzl JM, Hansen H. Structural competency and psychiatry. JAMA psychiatry 2018;75(2):115–6.
10. Hansen H, Metzl JM. New medicine for the US health care system: training physicians for structural interventions. Acad Med journal of the Association of American Medical Colleges 2017;92(3):279.
11. Hansen H, Metzl J. Structural competency in the US healthcare crisis: putting social and policy interventions into clinical practice. J Bioeth Inq 2016;13(2):179–83.

Part I

Structural Competency in Classrooms and Clinics

Teaching and Testing Structural Competency in Pre-health Undergraduate Classrooms

Jonathan M. Metzl, JuLeigh Petty, and Philip J. Pettis

The Problem

Racism and bias reside, not just in individual attitudes or interactions but within larger systems, structures, and institutions. For instance, calls for police sensitivity training in the aftermath of the 2014 police shooting of Michael Brown in Ferguson, Missouri, were exposed as insufficient when it became clear that racial tensions resulted not just from the attitudes of individual officers but from a series of structural factors. These included systemic racism in the police force [1], zoning rules that classified white neighborhoods as residential and black neighborhoods as commercial or industrial, urban renewal plans that shifted black populations from central cities like St. Louis to inner suburbs like Ferguson and segregated public housing projects that replaced integrated low-income areas [2].

These and other developments suggest how, when teaching healthcare providers and students about racism and bias in medicine, medical education needs to also conceptualize and intervene into forms of racism that physician and public health scholar Camara Jones describes as "structural, having been codified in our institutions of custom, practice, and law" and manifest through differential access to "the goods, services, and opportunities of society by race" [3]. Picking up this formulation, the White Coats for Black Lives movement calls for national medical school curricular standards that include "strategies for dismantling structural racism" [4].

To date, most structural competency interventions have targeted healthcare providers and medical students. However, our recent curricular efforts have aimed to assess whether structural competency training is beneficial in pre-health

J. M. Metzl (✉) · J. Petty
Center for Medicine, Health, and Society, Vanderbilt University, Nashville, TN, USA
e-mail: jonathan.metzl@vanderbilt.edu

P. J. Pettis
Department of Sociology, Vanderbilt University, Nashville, TN, USA

© Springer Nature Switzerland AG 2019

H. Hansen, J. M. Metzl (eds.), *Structural Competency in Mental Health and Medicine*,
https://doi.org/10.1007/978-3-030-10525-9_1

baccalaureate settings as well and in ways that potentially enhances how traditional premed education teaches students about diversity issues more broadly. Traditional pre-health education often separates pedagogy about the biological aspects of illness from training in other disciplines and approaches, with more emphasis on the former topics than on the latter ones [5]. A structural competency approach integrates scientific and medical advances with economics, sociology, anthropology, critical race studies, urban planning, epigenetics, and other frameworks in order to explore social and economic structures that contribute to inequities in the distribution of illnesses, as well as biases that surround attitudes about illness and health.

Theoretical Framework

Our focus on baccalaureate education rests in the belief that honing this kind of integrated knowledge during the undergraduate years becomes an ever more significant and applicable skill set for the next generation of health practitioners. Research increasingly uncovers how the pathologies of social and institutional systems impact the material realities of people's lives. Epigenetics, for instance, demonstrates at the level of gene methylation how high-stress, resource-poor environments can produce risk factors for disease that last for generations [6]. The MCAT now asks students to demonstrate aptitude in the influences of culture and community on health behaviors and outcomes, basics of the US healthcare system, social determinants of health, and changes in health policy [7, 8].

These and other developments suggest the importance of addressing matters such as race, culture, and bias through interdisciplinary pedagogic approaches that emphasize frameworks such as place, economy, politics, or history – a luxury not often afforded in oft-crowded professional school curricula. Despite increasing emphasis on the social foundations of health in premedical education, as recently as 2013–2014, less than half of all US universities and colleges offered an undergraduate course on health disparities [9].

The Path

In what follows, we briefly detail an interdisciplinary pre-health curriculum, the Medicine, Health, and Society (MHS) major at Vanderbilt University, that integrates structural competency frameworks into semester-long baccalaureate courses. We then discuss our published findings from an evaluation we undertook using a new evaluation tool, the Structural Foundations of Health Survey, that we developed to evaluate structural skills and sensibilities. Over a several year period, we used the survey to evaluate three groups of students at Vanderbilt University – incoming premed freshmen, graduating premed science majors, and graduating MHS majors – with particular attention to student analysis of how political, cultural, economic, and social factors such as institutional racism shape assumptions about conditions including cardiovascular disease, obesity, and depression.

We wondered whether MHS majors would identify and analyze relationships between structural factors and health outcomes in deeper ways than did premed science majors or incoming first-year students. And we wanted to know if MHS students also showed higher understandings of structural factors in their approaches to race, intersectionality, and health disparities. We also aimed to assess the value added of advanced instruction in structural approaches to race, racism, and inequity.

Medicine, Health, and Society

The Vanderbilt University pre-health major in Medicine, Health, and Society (MHS) combines coursework in health sciences, humanities, and social sciences. The MHS major emphasizes interdisciplinary study of health and illness in ways that encourage students to think critically about how complex social issues impact health, healthcare, and health policy.

Demand has been nothing short of remarkable. Enrollment rose from 40 students in 2008, to 160 students in 2009, to more than 300 students in 2012. By 2015 MHS enrolled over 500 undergraduate majors.

The authors of this chapter are the chair and assistant chair of MHS. In 2012–2013, we hosted a series of curricular redesign seminars for faculty in our unit, with the aim of reshaping the MHS curriculum in ways that emphasized respect for clinical advances alongside critical attention to the social, cross-cultural, racialized, and gendered determinants of health. Structural competency became the central unifying rubric in this curriculum. Faculty developed a number of structural competency-based interventions, including:

- A new course called Designing Healthy Publics studied how buildings, cities, and urban planning structure the health of populations.
- A new class on Community Health Research analyzed how health disparities are created and maintained by structural policies and practices.
- A number of classes on race, ethnicity, and health explored ways that historical, cultural, institutional, economic, and political factors shaped patterns of morbidity, food distribution networks, medication reimbursement rates, injury patterns, and other factors.
- Three new concentration areas (Intersectionality, Inequality, and Health Justice, Health Policies and Economies, Health Behaviors and Sciences) that combined pre-health science classes with courses that emphasized how cultural, economic, demographic, and biological factors impact health and two others (Global Health; Medicine, Humanities, and the Arts) that emphasized cross-cultural and literary structures of meaning.
- Structural immersion assignments added to medical humanities courses explored tensions between individual and social welfare in literary texts.
- Faculty-student colloquia that developed focus areas for classroom emphasis (e.g., structural understandings of race, health politics, critical analysis of representations of health).

Meanwhile, in-classroom assignments and activities were bolstered through course-related structurally competent immersion interventions such as:

- Service learning through placement in refugee resettlement agencies
- Student-provided Spanish translation services in low-income health clinics
- In-course emergency room rotations
- Attendance at legislative hearings on healthcare policy and the Affordable Care Act in Tennessee

Pertinent to this chapter, a majority of Vanderbilt students continued to pursue traditional pre-health degrees as pathways to professional schools. Most premed students majored in interdisciplinary sciences such as neuroscience, molecular and cellular biology, biomedical engineering, or other courses of study that emphasized life sciences along with smaller numbers of required general education courses in the humanities and social sciences [10].

The MHS-major medical school acceptance rate was higher than that of traditional pre-health science majors, and it was significantly higher than the national average. For instance, the 2016 medical school acceptance rates for applicants from the three most popular premedical majors at Vanderbilt were 72% for neuroscience, 78% for molecular and cellular biology, and 88% for MHS, compared to a national average of 42% [11].

Beneath the numbers, however, this divergence of two types of pre-health tracks at the same school – one (premed) that accentuated the traditional sciences and another (MHS) that promoted cultural and structural analysis alongside science prerequisites – allowed us to measure whether a curriculum based in structural competency might promote different analytic skills than did traditional premed tracks while at the same time preparing students for their post-college careers.

Structural Foundations of Health Survey

We next devised an evaluation instrument called the Structural Foundations of Health Survey [12–14] to assess and compare students' recognition of ways structural and institutional factors shape health outcomes. We crafted the instrument to try to capture awareness of health disparities and cultural differences, as well as structures and structural biases that produce them. We particularly emphasized core structural competency themes, including the ability to identify how economic, historical, and social conditions produce inequalities, rearticulate cultural differences in structural terms, recognize structural racism, and detect the ways that racial structures impact not just the health of minority populations but those of dominant groups.

The survey asked respondents about the underlying structural causes of conditions commonly attributed to lifestyle or biology: obesity, heart disease, and depression. This approach allowed assessment of the primary frameworks respondents used to understand inequalities in health. In response to critiques that most health disparities and cultural competency education focus on racial minorities in contrast to a white referent group [15], the survey also asked respondents to analyze depression based on an antidepressant advertisement featuring a white woman.

Our key findings are presented in full detail in a series of publications linked to this project. In brief, we collected data from graduating second-semester MHS-major seniors at Vanderbilt University in 2015 and 2016. We also collected data from two comparison groups at Vanderbilt: second-semester seniors not majoring or minoring in MHS who self-identified as planning careers in medicine ("premed seniors") and first-semester freshmen in their first 2 weeks of college who identified as planning careers in health professions. Key measures included the following.

Health Disparity-Related Professional Preparation

We measured students' self-reports of their awareness of health disparities and related professional preparation through four items on a 5-point scale ranging from poor (1) to excellent (5) preparation. Students self-reported their understanding of relationships between socioeconomic status (SES) and health, knowledge of the American health system, knowledge of the Affordable Care Act (ACA), and ability to work cooperatively with diverse populations. These areas of knowledge reflected the AAMC [16] "Core Competencies for Entering Medical Students."

Obesity

To assess structural competency, we asked participants to identify and explain geographic disparities in childhood obesity. We selected childhood obesity as an indicator of structural competency because explanations commonly invoke narratives of individual choice (lazy, weak will) or assumptions of deficiencies in culture and lifestyle instead of structural explanations such as food access [17]. The survey presented a map of the USA from the *Trust for America's Health* report in which the US South contained eight of the ten states with the highest rates of childhood obesity [18]. Participants were asked to select the three most important factors explaining this disparity from a list of 14 items that included individual-level factors (e.g., genetics, individual lifestyle choices), AAMC cultural competency factors (cultural background, health literacy, health traditions and beliefs, physician bias) [19], and structural competency factors as defined by Metzl and Hansen [20] (access to healthcare, health delivery system, insurance, institutional racism, medicalization, income, neighborhood, social policies).

Heart Disease

Next, we asked participants to explain a health disparity framed explicitly by race. We cited a statistic that, "African-American men are 30% more likely to die from heart disease than non-Hispanic white men" [21]. Here as well, presented closed- and open-ended questions to assess whether respondents phrased answers in relation to individual factors, "cultural" stereotypes about cardiovascular disease [22], or structural factors.

Depression

To detect student recognition of ways racial structures also potentially shape the health of privileged groups, we presented students with a pharmaceutical advertisement of an antidepressant ad showing a woman who appeared to be white who smiled while holding up a white-diapered infant above text that read, "I got my playfulness back!" The survey asked a series of open-ended questions: (1) "What is your initial response to this advertisement?" (2) "What messages does the advertisement convey about mental illness?" (3) "What role might social, political, economic, or cultural factors play in shaping the message of the advertisement?" Again, we coded individual versus structural factors, with particular attention to text regarding racial, cultural, or systemic understandings of mental illness.

Key Learnings

As expected, a majority of MHS seniors self-reported high levels of *health disparity-related professional preparation* including knowledge of the relationship between SES and health (95.1% excellent/good) and the US healthcare system (56.2% excellent/good). A substantial percentage also reported high levels of knowledge on the Affordable Care Act (48.1% excellent/good). These percentages were consistently higher than responses by premed seniors and first-year students ($p < 0.001$). MHS seniors also reported higher levels than premed seniors but not freshmen in preparation to work with diverse populations (74.6% versus 93.5%; t = $-4.225, p < 0.001$).

Analysis of the obesity and heart disease prompts supported these findings. MHS seniors were significantly more likely than the other groups of respondents to identify structural factors (e.g., neighborhood, access, health delivery system, institutional racism, income) to explain health inequalities. For instance, MHS seniors were over three times more likely than premed seniors to identify a structural factor as one of the three most important factors in explaining disparities in cardiac mortality (OR = 3.27, 95% CI = 1.37–7.82) and almost six times more likely to identify any structural factor as one of the three most important factors in explaining geographic disparities in childhood obesity (OR = 5.87, 95% CI = 2.89–11.92). In particular, MHS students were almost three times as likely as premed seniors to select institutional racism in response to the heart disease prompt (OR = 2.801, 95% CI = 1.565–5.105). Compared to premed seniors, MHS seniors were less likely to select an individual factor (e.g., lifestyle) to explain childhood obesity (OR = 0.412, 95% CI = 0.234–0.726) and equally likely to select an individual factor in the case of racial disparities in cardiac mortality.

We observed a strong, positive association between identification of structural factors that explained childhood obesity and cardiac mortality and number of MHS courses taken ($X^2 = 31.785$, $p < 0.001$). The identification of structural determinants of health for obesity and cardiac mortality significantly increased with the number of MHS courses taken by students in all groups. A majority (81%) of the students who did not identify any structural factors as one of the three most important determinants of cardiac mortality and childhood obesity had taken zero MHS courses.

Analysis of the depression prompt revealed that respondents in all groups were equally unlikely to identify or discuss structures that might enable privilege such as money, health insurance, or free time, when the object of analysis was a white woman. These numbers were consistently lower than those observed in the obesity or heart disease prompts, though by design we did not mention race or privilege in our formulation of any of the questions. Instead, we aimed to assess whether students would consider these factors without prompt, thereby reading against the "invisibility" of whiteness in the rhetorics surrounding health disparities [23]. Overall, compared to freshmen, MHS seniors were four times as likely to analyze SES (OR = 4.083, 95% CI = 1.767–9.432) and three times as likely to analyze whiteness (OR = 3.148, 95% CI = 1.464–6.772). We observed no significant differences between MHS and premed seniors.

Responses to open-ended prompts suggested deeper level differences between the three groups regarding the types of reasoning that students used to explain the relationships between structure, culture, and disparity/privilege. As predicted from the close-ended results, MHS responses more frequently linked structural and cultural explanations. Moreover, MHS seniors were less likely to reflect a monolithic view of African American culture. The most common themes in MHS students' cultural explanations included health seeking, trust, and lack of knowledge. Common attributes in non-MHS premed seniors and freshmen replies included monolithic African American culture, vagueness, and lack of knowledge.

For instance, non-MHS premed seniors and freshmen often assumed causal linkages in which monolithic culture (e.g., *their background*) produced unhealthy action (*tolerate more pain*) which then produced disease while at the same time assuming a unified, static notion of "African American" culture distinct from white culture or US culture. Typical responses to the cardiovascular and obesity questions included:

Perhaps the cultural norm is to try to tolerate more pain, including chest pain... (Premed senior #9)

There is more of a cultural influence on African American men than white men. The culture surrounding food intake is less healthy... (Premed senior #17)

Their background consists of slavery so they may eat less healthy food like biscuits and gravy... (Premed senior #3)

While some MHS students similarly assumed monolithic "culture" based on race ("African American men have poor health seeking behavior"), their responses frequently demonstrated added structural explanations to for cultural ones. For instance:

...residential segregation concentrates many black men in poor neighborhoods, where healthy foods and exercise facilities cannot be accessed, but where there are a lot of fast food restaurants. (MHS 2015 #42)

African American men are less likely to have health insurance than non-Hispanic white men...leads to males skipping yearly physicals and putting off seeing a doctor until symptoms are severe. (MHS 2016 #67)

To be sure, scholars [24, 25] have long associated culturally specific health beliefs and practices with expressions of illness. However, MHS students also demonstrated key structural competency components [20] including recognizing how structures shaped the social construct of disease, developing an extra-clinical language of structure, and rearticulating "cultural" formulations in structural terms.

MHS student explanations reflected the claim that health-seeking behavior is shaped by cultural beliefs, and they often referred to health seeking in relation to masculinity, distrust related to discrimination, and access:

African-American men may have less access to healthcare because they are less likely to visit a doctor and consequently less likely to be referred to specialists. In other words, institutional racism may prevent these men from being referred to these specialists which are essential in preventing and treating heart problems. Secondly, African American males tend to avoid going to the doctor because of cultural traditions of pride and strength, and health beliefs in which they do not like to show weakness...

Many black men do not have adequate health care, so it is not that they do not take care of their bodies as well as white men, but rather do not go the doctor as often as white men. The lack of trust of doctors also plays apart in black men's infrequent doctor visitations which is a result of history of abuse and misuse on the part of physicians...

No premed seniors or freshmen referenced health-seeking behaviors in structural terms.

Considerable differences regarding the role of genetics or genetic explanations of illness were seen among the three groups. Freshmen and premed non-MHS seniors often presented genetic explanations as causal in ways that directly explained morbidity and mortality of minority populations. Representative responses included:

African Americans men may be more susceptible to deadly consequences of heart disease due in part to their genetic makeup... (Freshman, #19)

Genetically African Americans have a higher incidence of developing heart failure at younger ages due to genetic factors such as high blood pressure and cholesterol... (Premed senior #43)

...genetic factors must play an important role in this because the difference is so high between african american and Caucasian. (Freshman, #60)

Some first-year students who provided genetic explanations in the open-ended responses also addressed lower individual income. However, these students rarely addressed large-scale social forces such as neighborhood, segregation, or food access.

Cultural difference often appeared as a correlate to genetics in these explanations in ways that seemed to amplify problems with approaching health disparities as a results of given characteristics shared by all members of a racial or ethnic group rather than as the outcome of underlying social processes,

> *Genetic issues like high bp are unique to some races. Lower literacy among AA males = less health literacy and knowledge about how to protect self, leading to low income = worse health and choices.* (Freshman, #8)

> *I think that there is a little bit of ignorance about food nutrition…different regions of the country have different genetics because many people grow up and stay in the same area, which limits the genetic pool.* (Premed senior #36)

MHS majors were considerably less likely than freshmen and premed seniors to argue that racial differences directly produced genetic components. Their responses often framed genetics within contexts of social or institutional factors of within caveats about the limits of genetic expertise:

> *Cultural background and genetic factors might create a genetic predisposition for heart disease in African American men. However, physicians may think of this statistic and jump to conclusions for African-American men when there is actually a deeper issue.* (MHS 2016 #55)

> *African American men may be more susceptible to deadly consequences of heart disease due in part to their genetic makeup but institutional racism may also play a part as African American men may be less likely to be diagnosed with heart disease, as compared to non-Hispanic white men.* (MHS 2015 #22)

MHS students were the only respondents who addressed epigenetic explanations for illness that articulated how social and environmental factors such as education, nutrition, history, or social conditions impacted genetic expression:

> *There is evidence to suggest that stress on pregnant mothers causes alterations in gene expression which are linked to higher rates of CVD later in life…* (MHS 2016 #7),

> *…genetics- stems from ancestors and their experiences with extreme racism, stress and strain on bodies…* (MHS 2015 #51)

Overall, our research suggested to us that students who graduated from an interdisciplinary pre-health curriculum (MHS) identified and analyzed relationships between structural factors and health outcomes at higher rates and in deeper ways than did premed science majors and first-term freshmen. While all groups demonstrated awareness of the impact of cross-cultural factors on health outcomes, MHS majors consistently demonstrated advanced skills that implied more nuanced understandings of structures underlying these outcomes. For instance, MHS students detailed structural or institutional disparities in complex ways and more commonly defined these disparities as arising from socioeconomic differences, discrimination, or policies that resulted in intended or unintended racial consequences. These types of analytic skills rose in all students in direct proportion to the number of MHS courses taken.

Meanwhile, non-MHS premed seniors were no more likely than were first-term freshmen to identify structural factors as causes of heart disease or obesity disparities. In the case of heart disease, premed non-MHS seniors were more likely than premed freshmen to identify a cultural (as opposed to structural) factor. These findings suggest that premed non-MHS seniors learned cultural skills but not structural ones as part of the premed curriculum, particularly in relationship to racial disparities.

Translation to Other Sites

To be sure, many schools cannot support the integrated, comprehensive structural health curriculum of Vanderbilt, which required recruitment of qualified faculty and institutional support for their collective pedagogical development efforts. Yet we hope our analysis suggests the salience of integrating structural frameworks into existing courses in order to more fully address structural disparities in addition to individual-level biases.

Our data further suggests that structural competency is a skill set that develops from training and that improving awareness about structural equity and well-being results not just from challenging students' implicit biases or sensitivities but from imparting analytic skills.

Of course, it may well be argued that MHS students simply reproduced the structural language and analysis emphasized by their coursework. But this is in part the point – the skills that these students demonstrated represent ones increasingly relevant, in an era of epigenetics, neighborhood effects, and social determinants, to address how contextual factors shape expressions of health and illnesses [26, 27]. Indeed, MHS students showed enhanced ability to "diagnose" issues such as structural determinants of health and structural stigma while at the same time also demonstrating deeper self-critical understandings of the "cultural" components of cultural competency.

Our research thus contributes to an evolving literature suggesting that teaching students about the "social" foundations of health needs to begin sooner in the educational process, during the baccalaureate years, when access to interdisciplinary pedagogies remains accessible, and when semester-long courses can promote frameworks that help future healthcare providers conceptualize links between health justice and social change.

References

1. The 12 key highlights from the DOJ's scathing Ferguson report – the Washington Post [Internet]. [cited 2018 Oct 1]. Available from: https://www.washingtonpost.com/news/post-nation/wp/2015/03/04/the-12-key-highlights-from-the-dojs-scathing-ferguson-report/?noredirect=on&utm_term=.626c9b5d0b80

2. The making of Ferguson: public policies at the root of its troubles [Internet]. Economic Policy Institute. [cited 2018 Oct 1]. Available from: https://www.epi.org/publication/making-ferguson/

3. Jones CP. Levels of racism: a theoretic framework and a gardener's tale. Am J Public Health. 2000;90(8):1212–5.

4. White Coats For Black Lives [Internet]. [cited 2018 Oct 1]. Available from: http://whitecoats-4blacklives.org/

5. Dalen JE, Alpert JS. Premed requirements: the time for change is long overdue! Am J Med. 2009;122(2):104–6.

6. Slopen N, Non A, Williams DR, Roberts AL, Albert MA. Childhood adversity, adult neighborhood context, and cumulative biological risk for chronic diseases in adulthood. Psychosom Med. 2014;76(7):481–9.

7. Association of American Medical Colleges. Behavioral and social science foundations for future physicians: report of the behavioral and social science expert panel. [document on the internet]. Washington, DC: Association of American Medical Colleges; 2011 Nov [cited 2015 Nov 6]. Available from: https://www.aamc.org/download/271020/data/behavioralandsocialsciencefoundationsforfuturephysicians.pdf

8. Association of American Medical College. Taking the MCAT® exam [document on the internet]. Washington, DC: Association of American Medical College; 2015 [cited 2015 Nov 6]. Available from: https://students-residents.aamc.org/applying-medical-school/taking-mcat-exam/

9. Benabentos R, Ray P, Kumar D. Addressing health disparities in the undergraduate curriculum: an approach to develop a knowledgeable biomedical workforce. CBE Life Sci Educ. 2014;13(4):636–40.

10. Baum R, Rains L. Health professions advisory office 2015 annual report of Vanderbilt University [document on the internet]. Nashville: Vanderbilt University; 2016 Jan 18 [cited 2018 Sept 25]. Available from: https://www.vanderbilt.edu/hpao/documents/2015_Annual_Report_2016-01-18.pdf

11. Grundy M, Rains L, Craion A. Health professions advisory office 2016 annual report of Vanderbilt University [document on the internet]. Nashville: Vanderbilt University; 2016 [cited 2017 Feb 1]. Available from: http://as.vanderbilt.edu/hpao/documents/2016_HPAO_Annual_Report-2017-01-30.pdf

12. Metzl JM, Petty J. Integrating and assessing structural competency in an innovative prehealth curriculum at Vanderbilt University. Acad Med. 2017;92(3):354–9.

13. Metzl JM, Petty J, Olowojoba OV. Using a structural competency framework to teach structural racism in pre-health education. Soc Sci Med. 2018;199:189–201.

14. Petty J, Metzl JM, Keys MR. Developing and evaluating an innovative structural competency curriculum for pre-health students. J Med Humanit. 2017;38(4):459–71.

15. Daniels SA. Constructing whiteness in health disparities research. In: Schulz AJ, Mullings L, editors. Health and illness at the intersections of gender, race and class. San Francisco: Jossey-Bass Publishing; 2006. p. 89–127.

16. Association of American Medical Colleges. Core competencies for entering medical students [document on the internet]. Washington, DC: Association of American Medical Colleges; 2014 [cited 2015 Nov 6]. Available from: https://www.staging.aamc.org/initiatives/admissionsinitiative/competencies/

17. Azzarito L. The rise of the corporate curriculum: fatness, fitness, and whiteness. In: Wright J, Harwood V, editors. Biopolitics and the 'obesity epidemic': governing bodies. 1st ed. New York: Routledge; 2008. p. 183–223.

18. Levi J, Vinter S, Laurent RS, Segal LM. F as in fat: how obesity policies are failing in America: 2007 [document on the internet]. Washington, DC: Trust for America's Health; 2008 [cited 2015 Nov 6]. Available from: http://healthyamericans.org/reports/obesity2009/
19. Association of American Medical Colleges. Cultural competence education [document on the internet]. Washington, DC: Association of American Medical Colleges; 2005 [cited 2015 Nov 6]. Available from: https://www.aamc.org/download/54338/data/
20. Metzl JM, Hansen H. Structural competency: theorizing a new medical engagement with stigma and inequality. Soc Sci Med. 2014;103:126–33.
21. U.S. Department of Health and Human Services. HHS action plan to reduce racial and ethnic health disparities: implementation progress report 2011–2014 [document on the internet]. Washington, DC: U.S. department of Health and Human Services; 2014 [cited 2015 Nov 16]. Available from: http://minorityhealth.hhs.gov/assets/pdf/FINAL_HHS_Action_Plan_Progress_Report_11_2_2015.pdf
22. Pollock A. Medicating race: heart disease and durable preoccupations with difference. Durham: Duke University Press; 2012.
23. Sue DW. Whiteness and ethnocentric monoculturalism: making the "invisible" visible. Am Psychol. 2004;59(8):761–9.
24. James D. Factors influencing food choices, dietary intake, and nutrition-related attitudes among African Americans: application of a culturally sensitive model. Ethn Health. 2004;9(4):349–67.
25. Airhihenbuwa CO, Kumanyika S, Agurs TD, Lowe A, Saunders D, Morssink CB. Cultural aspects of African American eating patterns. Ethn Health. 1996;1(3):245–60.
26. Robert Wood Johnson E. A new way to talk about the social determinants of health [document on the internet]. Robert wood Johnson Foundation; 2011; [cited 2015 Nov 6]. Available from: http://www.rwjf.org/content/dam/farm/reports/reports/2010/rwjf63023
27. Goldstein D, Jaclyn, H. Health and wellness survey: 2011 Physicians' Daily Life Poll. Harris interactive [document on the internet]; 2011 Nov 15 [cited 2015 Nov 6]. Available from: http://www.rwjf.org/content/dam/web-assets/2011/11/2011-physicians%2D%2Ddaily-life-report. Accessed 6 Nov 2015.

The Walking Classroom and the Community Clinic: Teaching Social Medicine Beyond the Medical School

Jeremy A. Greene, Graham Mooney, and Carolyn Sufrin

Many medical students already feel as if they understand the social determinants of disease: a list of gradients in which it is worse to be on one end than the other. Poverty is associated with worse outcomes, check. Being part of a racial, ethnic, or linguistic minority is associated with worse outcomes, check. What more is there to learn? Moreover, what can the physician-in-training do beyond adopting the casual fatalism that it sucks to be poor, it's easier to be born white than black in America, and the deck is stacked against you if you are born into a non-English-speaking family? Give me something I can actually intervene on, they often say, like a blocked coronary artery or a fracture to repair, not these structural forces that physicians are powerless to change.

Over the past 5 years, we have offered a 6-week elective curriculum, "Introduction to Social Medicine," which takes first-year students out of the classroom and into East Baltimore. The aim is for students to learn fundamental theoretical, methodological, and pragmatic insights from social sciences to extend their understanding of the day-to-day factors driving health, illness, relapse, and recovery. This chapter

J. A. Greene (✉)
Department of the History of Medicine, Center for Medical Humanities and Social Medicine, Johns Hopkins University School of Medicine, Baltimore, MD, USA
e-mail: jgree115@jhmi.edu

G. Mooney
Institute of the History of Medicine, Center for Medical Humanities and Social Medicine, Johns Hopkins University School of Medicine, Department of Epidemiology, Baltimore, MD, USA

C. Sufrin
Department of Gynecology and Obstetrics, Center for Medical Humanities and Social Medicine, Johns Hopkins School of Medicine, Baltimore, MD, USA

Department of Health, Behavior and Society, Johns Hopkins Bloomberg School of Public Health, Baltimore, MD, USA

© Springer Nature Switzerland AG 2019   15
H. Hansen, J. M. Metzl (eds.), *Structural Competency in Mental Health and Medicine*,
https://doi.org/10.1007/978-3-030-10525-9_2

focuses on two of these initiatives—the walking classroom and the community clinic—to illustrate how these tactics can be used by medical educators in a variety of different settings. These experiences are intended to help students learn to practice differently and to see structural determinants of health and disease as central parts of the medical encounter that they can do something about: equally important to diagnose, prognose, and intervene upon as a blocked coronary artery.

The Problem: Placing Social Medicine in the Curriculum

Who gets sick, who gets better, and why? When treatments of known efficacy are available, why do they fail so often? Who or what causes a patient to be nonadherent with their treatment plan? All physicians encounter such questions in their clinical work. They are questions of social medicine, a field of inquiry that uses the methods of the social sciences and the humanities to analyze how disease and medicine unfold in the lives of real people living in real places. As the physician and historian George Rosen noted in 1948, this "idea of medicine as a social science" [1] was an essential part of the development of modern medicine.

Despite this, only a handful of North American medical schools contain departments of social medicine (Harvard Medical School [2], the University of North Carolina [3], the University of California San Francisco [4], Ohio University [5], and Albert Einstein College of Medicine [6]). Although some of these schools mount a robust social science curriculum, the bulk produce at best a fragmented sense of how physicians can learn about and intervene in the social worlds of their patients.

This is partly an unintended consequence of medical education reform in the early twenty-first century, which has focused on compressing the preclinical curriculum, shifting courses to integrated modules, and emphasizing the "competencies" that physicians should be expected to demonstrate. On the one hand, this approach has "vertical" strands of integrated modules based on organ systems and on the other hand "vertical" strands in which the social basis of medical care will be taught. But in practice, the coordination of these strands tends to be haphazard and often nonexistent. At Johns Hopkins, for example, the most recent integrative reform took place in 2009, with the launch of the "Genes to Society" curriculum [7]. Though this title reflects a noble attempt to include the vast range of social and biological elements of medical education, the two are not given equal weight. "Genes" are taught in every main block of the preclinical curriculum, from the first (Scientific Foundations of Medicine) through the last (reproductive/musculoskeletal). "Society," on the other hand, gets subsumed into scattered modules on "Health Care Disparities" and "Cultural Competence," as a perfunctory addition to other lecture slides, or emerges as aspirational themes for course directors to incorporate.

We describe here an alternative approach which takes students out of the classroom altogether and brings them into neighborhoods and a community clinic in order to learn directly from people and institutions that constitute the social worlds that determine patients' health, as a first step toward fostering community-engaged clinical practice.

Theoretical Framework

"Introduction to Social Medicine" was launched in the fall of 2013 and has slowly built ranks from a handful of students the first year to a sizeable number of self-selected first-year medical students. The course, delivered in 8 h over 6 weeks, makes a case for the value of social sciences in preclinical education. While there are many disciplinary frameworks through which to teach social and structural forces shaping health and healthcare, we used social medicine as our approach for its interdisciplinary nature and for the ways it lends itself to translation into clinically meaningful lessons for students developing their sense of professional selves.[1] The first 3 weeks introduce students to the theory and practice of social medicine, including case studies and readings in structural violence and the social determinants of health, to enable them to recognize these forces wherever they work, to understand how they affect their patients, and to develop appropriate responses. We emphasize scalar continuities between local and global, showing how insights gained in one setting can often be applied and adapted in many others. Our pedagogical approach also encourages students to question their assumptions about patients, treatments, hospital systems, and other taken for granted concepts like cultural competence, and this sense of critique is incorporated into classroom and out of classroom learning.

Sessions are designed to be dynamic and case-based, combining a small lecture with an interactive tutorial. The latter sessions relate these general principles to Baltimore City. The course situates medical students' education beyond the Johns Hopkins academic medical center and into the East Baltimore neighborhoods where their patients live. This geographic specificity serves not only to increase their familiarity with their patients' surrounding environment but also to push them to consider the complex relationship between Johns Hopkins as an institution and the people and neighborhoods in which it is embedded. Students are challenged to rethink their approach to the "social history" and to consider social resources not included in most medical textbooks when caring and advocating for patients in their future clinical careers [8].

---

[1] The term "social medicine" has been adopted and developed in a variety of ways. By social medicine, we mean the understanding of how health, disease and medical care are determined by social and economic factors, and the ways in which that knowledge can be implemented to foster healthier outcomes.

The Approach I: The Walking Classroom

The walking classroom stresses the importance of understanding social determinants of health as a changing set of forces that can be studied, whose directionality and relevance are not necessarily knowable ahead of time and whose elucidation can lead to real possibilities for change and advocacy. In a two-part tutorial, we examine health inequalities in Baltimore neighborhoods, try to understand possible social determinants, and imagine possible interventions or solutions. This project draws on the Baltimore City Health Department's (BCHD) neighborhood health reports for community statistical areas, which contain basic demographic information and measures of life expectancy, mortality, morbidity, risk factors, food availability, etc. Our attention focuses on three neighborhoods close to the Hopkins medical campus, Madison/East End, Patterson Park N&E, and Fells Point, which, while they share geographic proximity to Johns Hopkins, differ on many sociodemographic measures.

Cartographically, the socioeconomic, racial, and health inequalities of Baltimore appear stark, with a sharp demarcation between self-identifying African-American and self-identifying white residents. Health disparities can be traced by following high/low gradients from neighborhood to neighborhood, such as the 17-year difference in life expectancy at birth in 2013 between Cross Country/Cheswolde in the north (85.3 years) and Madison/East End (68.2 years) by the Hopkins medical campus [9] [Fig. 2].

Students work in small teams and pick a category of health or disease, such as HIV/AIDS, cancer, heart disease, or suicide, and note its distribution across the three neighborhoods. Using demographic and socioeconomic data in the reports, students hypothesize their understandings of how these places and their health profiles can be related. Quickly, the students begin to grapple with the fact that not all forms of disease move along the same socioeconomic gradients; the social determinants of disease take on more complexity and become sites of potential agency and advocacy, rather than fatalism (as noted below in student observations on lead paint poisoning and vacant properties).

The next week takes students on a walking route from the medical school, through Madison/East End, via Patterson Park N&E, to upper Fells Point. Students are asked to notice what they learn at street level. What observations simply corroborate the data they analyzed previously? How do boundary lines drawn on a map obfuscate transitions or emphasize differences between neighborhoods? What speaks to lack, need, failure of infrastructure, and decay, and what speak to assets, capital in all its forms, community cohesion, resources, and strengths? And where is all this still not enough? What more do they wish they knew about in order to better understand the social determinants of health or intervene on behalf of their patients? Students then write an essay summarizing their observations and reflections on these questions.

Student responses are telling. Take, for example, this exploration of diet, health, and chronic disease:

Residents in Patterson Park have the shortest estimated travel time to a supermarket (4-minute walk) compared to Fells Point and Middle East (10 and 15-minute walks respectively). Middle East has the highest density of corner stores, while Fells Point has the least and Fells point has the highest density of fast food restaurants, while Patterson Park has the least.

... Residents of Patterson Park, despite having seemingly high access to supermarkets have the highest incidence of deaths related to heart disease. In Middle East, the high density of corner stores may be in place to fill the gaps that a lack of supermarkets creates, but typically these corner stores are unable to stock a sufficient produce selection. Fells Point residents also have a relatively far walk to a supermarket and have a high density of fast food and corner stores—all indicating a poor food environment—yet the residents have the lowest incidence of deaths associated with chronic disease.

... the inconsistencies raise a number of questions ... between the picture that the numbers portray and what residents actually may be experiencing; this "urban transect geography" provides insight into some of the confounding variables that influence dietary behaviors and health.

The discrepancy between prediction and data was, in and of itself, valuable for this student to understand that health phenomena are complex and cannot be understood in a statistical vacuum. Students are also encouraged to reflect on alternative ways of knowing these communities: journalism, history, sociology, ethnography, and community engagement. As another student described, after being troubled by the substantial disparities in high levels of childhood lead poisoning:

In the health profile study, lead paint violation rates for Middle East was significantly worse than the Baltimore City average, with Patterson Park being almost on par and Fells Point being significantly better ... Baltimore City's seeming disregard for vacant housing and neighborhood development in the Middle East could surely contribute to the frequency of lead paint violations in existing housing. In Fells Point, where vacant housing is less common, the attention of homeowners as well as developers to the neighborhood would unsurprisingly result in checks to prevent lead poisoning in homes.

The recognition of such diverse, intersecting factors might be crippling, at first, in searching for solutions to the health disparity between the Middle East and Fells Point. If lead poisoning contributes to poor education outcomes *as well as* health outcomes, efforts should be made by the city to enact housing development policies that allow housing in the neighborhood to be both *livable* and affordable for people in the neighborhood ... but the structural issues at play for health disparities in Baltimore's neighborhood requires more than an effort by physicians – it requires a city wide push by politicians, realtors, community leaders, and more.

Most responses contain a sense of the limitations of the assignment: after all, how much can one learn from 2 h walk through three neighborhoods? But they also reflect a critical sensibility of the utility and limitations of the data published by BCHD and desire to go beyond clinical care in order to address the health inequalities described by the data.

The walking classroom has received high ratings from students. Yet in its first years, when the module was presented as a "tour" and not a "walking classroom," students gave voice to some discomfort. Indeed, the author of the quote above also identified the faculty instructor as "our tour guide." Some suggested that perhaps the "research" that they were conducting on social determinants of health should require IRB approval and a signed informed consent form from any "subjects" that they spoke with. Others noted the problems with calling it a "tour":

> I'm a little conflicted about the walking tour of Baltimore. While I understand the purpose of it and think it is useful in getting a little more familiar with the context of the neighborhoods around Hopkins, there is an element of "poverty tourism" that runs through it that I'm not entirely comfortable with. Part of it I think has to do with how conspicuous we are as a group (I wonder if it's feasible to do the tour in smaller groups, for instance?) so it's clear that we are literally on a tour observing the neighborhoods around us; I think part of it is also that the tour is still led by Hopkins faculty/affiliates and there isn't an effort to engage with non-Hopkins members of these communities, so that it becomes an exercise of us projecting our readings onto these people and places. I'm honestly not quite sure what would work better, but I think at least more attention to these dynamics and thinking about how to make the tour less of a "tour" would be helpful.

The module is designed as neither research nor tourism: it is intended to be a form of experiential education outside the classroom, informed by pedagogical theory and practice. Our students live in each of the three neighborhoods we discuss; our patients are drawn from each of them as well; our academic medical center sits at their intersection. To walk through these streets is not to gawk, point, be amused, or conduct research, but to acknowledge the continuity and change in the different parts of the city we all inhabit. Yet the module does need to be carefully built to avoid the perils of seeing the neighborhoods of East Baltimore as some sort of "living laboratory" for Johns Hopkins University, on the one hand, or a form of student tourism on the other [10]. As the module has developed, we have worked to emphasize, above all, that community engagement itself is neither research nor tourism: it is an aspect of civic life and an opportunity to participate. More recent student evaluations have been uniformly sanguine about the experience, rating it as unambiguously positive: "I really liked the walking classroom"; "It taught us to shift the paradigm"; for one student, it highlighted the possibilities of "Being able to go into the community and apply theory to practice" [11]. In the class after the walking classroom, we then engage students in discussions about how their observations and insights might come to bear in clinical settings.

The Approach II: The Clinic and Its Communities

Like many academic medical centers, Johns Hopkins has a history of fractious relations with the communities that live closest to its doors, something which students hear about formally and informally throughout their preclinical and clinical years.

A contentious conversation over whether the presence of the school and hospital helps or harms its closest neighbors has persisted from the construction of the initial hospital in the late nineteenth century up to the school's present involvement in the ambitious East Baltimore Development Initiative [12]. Even as the academic medical center responded to the 2015 Freddie Gray uprising with new initiatives such as Baltimore CONNECT, a project to "build capacity among the community organizations and improve the health outcomes for East Baltimore and Southeast Baltimore residents," [13] many local residents still colloquially refer to the medical center as "the plantation," "the octopus," or "the elephant," [14] with personal histories of experimentation and exploitation all too fresh in living memory [15, 16].

The views of residents toward a local community health center run by Johns Hopkins, the East Baltimore Medical Center (EBMC), are not quite as monolithic. Set in the middle of row homes and housing projects in the Middle East neighborhood, northwest of the academic medical center and adjacent to the city's sprawling jail complex, EBMC is a very different site to learn about the engagement of a clinic with its multiple communities.

This module situates the community health center as a site for learning about the social determinants of health and disease, the social structures in which patients seek care and treatment, and the kinds of interventions available for individuals and populations. It also encourages students to question their assumptions about what community means and how the concept is deployed in clinical settings. The 2-h block is divided into another walking classroom (this time indoors), followed by a discussion of the changing structure of the community healthcare center and the multiple communities it serves.

Students are first asked to notice what surrounds the clinic as they enter—row homes, churches, a jail. The bulk of the module is led by a care coordinator in the department of medicine, a local resident with a long institutional memory, who can trace a personal history of medical care in the clinic since shortly after her own birth: from her first pediatric visits to her current primary care physician. Her tour connects the main sections of the community health center through the back doors: internal medicine, OB/GYN, pediatrics, dentistry, urgent care, and key ancillary services (social work, patient registration, administration, pharmacy, laboratory, radiology). Waiting rooms house a mix of patients, some from the nearby row homes and public housing, others local employees of Johns Hopkins, still others from a further-flung set of Baltimore neighborhoods who come for EBMC's safety-net assistance programs and/or its Spanish-speaking practitioners. Enlarged photos on the walls of each division feature faces from the community; our guide pauses to point out a particularly well-framed photograph of her father, working as a local medical assistant in the mid-1970s. Near the front entrance hang paintings of three prominent founders of the clinic: local African-American politicians from city and state government who were crucial to its construction and who formed part of the initial governing board.

After the narrated walk through the clinic, we then gather students into a conference room at the health center to discuss the history of EBMC's contentious beginnings, using newspaper archives. The health center was opened in 1971 as a direct result of negotiations between Johns Hopkins, the City of Baltimore, and prominent members of the East Baltimore community in the immediate aftermath of the April 1968 riots. It was notable as the first self-covered community health center of its kind, offering residents care through the East Baltimore Medical Plan, a federally financed but community-owned prepaid medical plan available to any person receiving Medicare, Medicaid, children or youth funds, or similar aid from federal, state, or municipal agencies [17]. The communities and the center have changed in many ways since then, but the question of *which* community the health center was designed to serve was fractious, even at the planning stage [18]. African-American activists from West Baltimore protested the East Baltimore Community Corporation as an unrepresentative sham. Vocal East Baltimore residents, in turn, critiqued their West Baltimore counterparts for meddling. By the early 1980s, federal funding mechanisms of the East Baltimore Medical Plan ended under the new fiscal realities of the Reagan administration. Johns Hopkins and private funding organizations then intervened and EBMC was consolidated as merely one of several locations for the Johns Hopkins Community Physicians—a network of practices designed as "feeders" for the academic medical center.

Using historical newspaper articles, the personal history of their local guide, conversations with practitioners and staff, and observations on the functioning of the clinic today, the students are tasked with understanding the communities the clinic now serves. They explore the relationship of EBMC's daily functions relative to the original goals of the clinic. The students have discovered that as the structure has changed, the cohesion of the parts has lessened. The pharmacy, now operated as a Rite-Aid franchise, charges high prices for off-patent drugs. The dental clinic will not see Medicaid patients. The OB/GYN clinic is a semiprivate practice which is generally unavailable for urgent care ultrasonography. The on-site radiology clinic is only open at limited hours. And yet most of the practitioners working at EBMC do so out of a sense of the possibility to provide better care to the local communities of East Baltimore—a sense shared by all of us. Many of the Center's primary care physicians share an institutional memory reaching back to the original goals. Staff and social workers ensure EBMC is a place where undocumented Latino patients from across the city, and local residents recently discharged from the nearby city jail, find affordable care and do not slip between the healthcare system's cracks.

Students universally rated this session highly: "I love love loved the chance to have conversations about questions in medicine that can't be answered with experiments," said one of them. Most had never been inside of a community health center before, and none had had a sustained chance to understand the built structure of the clinic as a product of social and political action, imprinted with the grand social designs of and social conflicts of the 1960s, reshaped in the alternating political and economic moments of the 1980s and 1990s, to be partially restored as a vehicle for reimagining healthcare in the twenty-first century. As another student mentioned, the session was a chance to explore how the spaces in which we provide care are a form of ruins, the shadow, perhaps, of the aspirations that prior generations of healthcare providers and communities hoped they would be, but a vital space for advocacy and action nonetheless.

Outcomes and Lessons Learned

In addition to these walking classrooms, other sessions of the course include small group discussion of patient vignettes; a peeling away of the theoretical layers in the concentric model of the social determinants of health which represents inherent factors such as age, sex, and genetics at the center, then layers of individual "lifestyle" determinants (e.g., smoking, exercise), social and community factors, and living and working conditions, and an outer layer of the broad general social, economic, and political variables [19][2]; and in-class exercises focused on the meaning and application of "cultural competence" and "cultural humility." These components come and go, depending on faculty expertise, faculty availability, and student evaluations.

As yet, we have not conducted any formal "before" and "after" measurements of student knowledge and learning. As with most other educational interventions, we rely on retrospective surveys of students, and these are standardized across the first-year program of electives in public health, health policy, and ethics, of which social medicine is but one.

Effective evaluation of the elective is restricted in other ways. Many—though by no means all—of the students taking this short course in social medicine are self-selecting. The format and duration of the course change year-by-year, making longitudinal assessment difficult. Nor is the student experience immersive. In the matrix of geographical fieldwork pedagogy, students practice a form of "dependent observation"—that is, they are dependent on faculty directing their inquiries and they observe phenomena through textual and visual sources—with little time to develop either participatory activities or ideas for autonomous projects.

Nonetheless, evaluations have been revealing. Students are keenly aware that using the city as a classroom is complex and needs to be handled carefully. This is a commonly understood phenomenon in the social sciences—such as geography and anthropology, where "the field" is often the site of study—but perhaps needs further contemplation when it is practiced in a discipline that is so conditioned to actively intervene in people's lives. Such sensitivity is particularly relevant in East Baltimore, where Johns Hopkins is viewed unfavorably by some, if not many, local residents.

Having said that, even the less enthusiastic student responses have acknowledged the limits under which the course has been constructed. Any time spent learning outside of the traditional classroom has been seen as valuable. The course has proved useful as one way of introducing a deeper theoretical background to engagement with the local community through student-led organizations. Thus, while most of these organizations existed prior to the introduction of the social medicine course, we now have a cohort of senior students who work with such organizations and

---

[2] There are multiple iterations of this model, many of which have been adapted for specific medical conditions. In this class, we use the original and probably most widely used version that first appeared in Gören Dahlgren and Margaret Whitehead, 1991. *Policies and Strategies to Promote Social Equity in Health*. Stockholm: Institute for Futures Studies.

return to the social medicine class and reaffirm its value to current students. Such outcomes have convinced us that a more cohesive framework is needed for putting the "social" into the Genes to Society curriculum at Hopkins and into medical education more generally. It is only a beginning: ideally a broader structural competency curriculum would include interprofessional training alongside nursing students and other allied healthcare personnel and would extend into the clinical years, internships, and residency structures as well. It is not that hard to imagine a model of medical education that takes these forms of engagement as seriously as we take dissection, microbiology, or genomics: as a set of broader opportunities that could allow community engagement to impact the trajectory of future physicians and vice versa.

Acknowledgments We would like to express our gratitude to the Johns Hopkins medical students who have participated in the Social Medicine elective and have provided valuable feedback on our efforts. We also are grateful to Arnetra Mercer at the East Baltimore Medical Center and to Eric Bass and Brenda Zacharko for their support and encouragement.

References

1. Rosen G. Approaches to a concept of social medicine; a historical survey. Milbank Mem Fund Q. 1948;26(1):7–21.
2. Department of Global Health & Social Medicine | [Internet]. [cited 2018 Oct 2]. Available from: http://ghsm.hms.harvard.edu/
3. Department of Social Medicine [Internet]. [cited 2018 Oct 2]. Available from: https://www.med.unc.edu/socialmed
4. Department of Anthropology, History and Social Medicine. [Internet]. [cited 2018 Oct 2]. Available from: http://dahsm.ucsf.edu/
5. Social Medicine. [Internet]. [cited 2018. Oct 2]. Available from: https://www.ohio.edu/medicine/about/departments/social/
6. Department of Family and Social Medicine. [Internet]. [cited 2018. Oct 2]. Available from: http://www.einstein.yu.edu/departments/family-social-medicine/
7. Wiener CM, Thomas PA, Goodspeed E, Valle D, Nichols DG. "Genes to society" – the logic and process of the new curriculum for the Johns Hopkins University School of Medicine. Acad Med. 2010;85(3):498–506.
8. Panelli R, Welch RV. Teaching research through field studies: a cumulative opportunity for teaching methodology to human geography undergraduates. J Geogr High Educ. 2005;29(2):255–77.
9. Baltimore City Health Department. Life expectancy in Baltimore City, 2013 [Internet]. [cited 2018 Oct 3]. Available from: https://health.baltimorecity.gov/sites/default/files/Life-expectancy-2013.pdf
10. Tracy SJ. Qualitative research methods: collecting evidence, crafting analysis, communicating impact. 1st ed. Chichester, West Sussex: Wiley-Blackwell; 2013.
11. Phillips R, Johns J. Fieldwork for human geography. 1st ed. London: SAGE Publications Ltd; 2012.
12. Gomez MB. Race, class, power, and organizing in East Baltimore: rebuilding abandoned communities in America. Lanham: Lexington Books; 2015.
13. Baltimore CONNECT – Affiliated Programs – Research – Johns Hopkins Bloomberg School of Public Health [Internet]. [cited 2018 Oct 2]. Available from: https://www.jhsph.edu/research/affiliated-programs/baltimore-connect/

14. Johns Hopkins Hospital inspires mistrust and fear in parts of East Baltimore – The Washington Post [Internet]. [cited 2018 Oct 2]. Available from: https://www.washing-tonpost.com/local/johns-hopkins-hospital-inspires-mistrust-and-fear-in-parts-of-east-baltimore/2017/01/25/a4f402c2-bbf3-11e6-91ee-1adddfe36cbe_story.html?noredirect=on&utm_term=.18b4670f559d

15. Markowitz G, Rosner D. Lead wars: The politics of science and the fate of America's children. 1st ed. Berkeley/New York: University of California Press; 2013.

16. Skloot R. The immortal life of Henrietta Lacks. New York: Broadway Books; 2011.

17. East Baltimore medical program to begin soon. The Baltimore Sun, September 12, 1971: A23.

18. Health Unit is proposed—but East Baltimore meeting opposes Hopkins plan. Baltimore Sun, October 2, 1969.

19. Dahlgren G, Whitehead M. Policies and strategies to promote social equity in health. Background document to WHO – Strategy paper for Europe. Institute for Futures Studies, Arbetsrapport. 1991: 14.

This Ain't No Tool, This Ain't No Toolbox

Edgar Rivera Colón

Preamble: This essay is a critical literary approach to structural competency which uses as its starting point the lives and thinking of figures from the Black Freedom movement as political role models for students in medical education. A premise of this essay is that professional training tends to depoliticize medical students and mold them into technical experts, but not necessarily freedom-minded civic and political activists. The crisis in the professions that we are witnessing with the advent of Trumpism is a challenge to the integrity of all professions and credentialing institutions like medical schools. The facile answer is call for professional neutrality. Structural competency can never be politically neutral in a society that is quickly moving to deeper divisions and open social conflict. This essay is a literary experiment in calibrating the ethical and political costs of training students at looking at medicine and its array of institutions from a conflict-based perspective. At the core of this essay are two underlying ethical questions: Will the healthcare professions be explicit and conscious about the political power they wield already? Also, what will they do with the power in these times of profound conflict?

Structural competency or the ability to discern and act to correct the ways health outcomes also represent the results of systemic institutional violence and exclusion is a critically important component of healthcare education to teach students structural competency is to invite them into the conflict of structural inequity and the difficult process of self-examination. But structural competency cannot simply be a new content area in healthcare curricula; it needs to represent a fundamental shift in pedagogical methods and instructional posture. The classroom, and thus the instructor, must reflect the collectivity and power-sharing that we expect our students to reflect and enact in their patient interactions. Infusing structural competence into

E. Rivera Colón (✉)
Narrative Medicine Program, Columbia University, New York, NY, USA

Saint Peter's University, The Jesuit University of New Jersey, Jersey City, NJ, USA
e-mail: ec2648@columbia.edu

© Springer Nature Switzerland AG 2019
H. Hansen, J. M. Metzl (eds.), *Structural Competency in Mental Health and Medicine*,
https://doi.org/10.1007/978-3-030-10525-9_3

medical education in classroom, community, and clinical spaces means inviting our students into a deeper sense of political and social responsibility as the beginning of a larger process of individual and collective self-development. This essay shares my experiences and pedagogical methods of slowing down, turning inward, and creating collective spaces of knowledge sharing in classrooms that enable our students to explore structural competency not simply as curricular content, but as a transformative personal experience. Fundamentally, this requires the deliberate action on the part of educators to reflect structural competency not only in our syllabi, but as an engaged and embodied process within ourselves.

> I did not come here to comfort you. I came here to disturb you. James Boggs

In November of 1963, at one of the many turning points that would put in stark relief the tensions between "integrationist" and "liberationist" tendencies in the Black Freedom Movement of the 1960s and 1970s, the Detroit-based autoworker, militant labor organizer, and community activist, James Boggs, addressed a meeting at New York City's Town Hall with the following words: "Now I did not come here to comfort you. I came here to disturb you. I did not come here to pacify you. I came here to antagonize you. I did not come here to talk to you about love. I came here to talk to you about conflict. I say this at the outset because the American people have lived for so long under the illusion that America is an exception to the deep crises that wreck other countries – that they are totally unprepared to face the brutish realities of the present crisis and the dangers that threaten them. The American people have lived so long with the myth that the United States is a Christian, capitalist, free democratic nation that we can do no wrong, that the question of what is right and wrong completely evades us" ([1], pp. 315–16).

Boggs grew up in Jim Crow Alabama and migrated before World War II, joining so many of his fellow African Americans in Northern cities, like Detroit, to work in the auto plants of the Motor City. He understood from bitter experience and long reflection on the many social struggles he participated in throughout his life the insulation from reality that white supremacy provides so many Americans then and now. His opening remarks during his 1963 speech were an attempt to awaken his audience to the brutal – and ofttimes bloody – realities of those on the bottom of the American social system and the general violence that delimits the life chances of the peoples of what we now call the Global South. Boggs was pushing his fellow activists, who gathered from across many organizations and points of view for this event, to be attentive to and centered in the main currents of the USA and world history as they strategized their next steps in the fight for freedom in 1960's America.

Clearly, this fight for freedom remains unfinished to our common peril and potential national and planetary ruin. The fact that Boggs's comments appear all too painfully relevant at our own historical moment in the wake of Donald Trump's election victory is evidence of how the "real existing" neoliberal political economies and racial formations we suffer under and endure now have *reconstituted*, not abolished, the social contradictions discussed during that Town Hall meeting more than 50 years ago [2]. What, then, are we doing when we begin to call upon our students to think and be *structurally competent* about the problems and challenges they face in their medical training and as future clinicians?

More to the point: are we, as educators, ready to do this work and what methods should we be using? In one sense, the raison d'etre of this volume is to provide concrete examples by which our students can operationalize – what Marx in his 1861–63 Notebooks (*Grundrisse*) would call the "concrete in thought" or the "concrete totality" – the call that Metzl and Hansen have initiated to find an "extra-clinical" language to name and intervene in the inequalities that make our communities sick and fill our emergency rooms and clinics every day ([3], p. 53, my translation; cite [4] paper SSM). To use Boggs's language, teaching students structural competency is to "disturb" and "antagonize" them and to invite them into "conflict" that render good intentions and facile renditions of "love" as sentiment mute before the ubiquitous, malevolent effects of structural violence and social exclusion.

When Audre Lorde wrote "The master's tools will never dismantle the master's house," [5] she was speaking of the ways of socially just change. She was speaking of revolution. Yet, in this era of corporate-speak, "tools" and "toolboxes" have come to stand for easily quantifiable and transferable skill sets, checkboxes of knowledge, and learner "competence." Like cultural competency training in health education, structural competency is burdened with medical education's terminology of preference, its predilection for measurable competencies. And yet, structural competency can and must be more than yet another tool in the healthcare practitioner's metaphoric toolbox.

The challenge of creating learning communities well-versed in structural competence and poised for action in medical education settings is largely a question of method and process, decidedly not a product or deliverables or even learning outcomes (notwithstanding our dean-mandated, ever-more detailed syllabi templates), if we wish to be sober in our assessment of the work ahead. To invite our students into the disturbing antagonisms of institutional and social conflicts – and that is the call we are making – is to leave the realm of epistemology and enter the social field or ontological landscape of transformative action in the service of health justice. That is no small order. If truth be told, it is a call to another way of life and immersion in a decades-long struggle to discover other more fruitful and just ways to flourish, occupy, and expand what we might become 1 day: human beings.

Slowing Down: The Question of Time

I chose to begin this essay with a quote by James Boggs because he elected to spend most of his adult life participating in struggles around labor rights, the Black Freedom Movement, the anti-war movement, urban education reform, and the women's liberation movement, and, toward the very end of his life, he helped initiate a Detroit Summer program that would bring older African Americans, many of whom had grown up in Southern farming communities, and young people together to build large gardens that would teach all involved the value of collective work, reflection on that work, and the exercise of new social imaginaries through which abandoned urban lots becomes the economic and social infrastructure for a new Detroit as well as an alternative to rapacious displacement of working-class communities of color via gentrification and real estate speculation in many of our urban centers.

Boggs never stopped asking questions, accounting for his errors in analysis and judgment, or posing new ways to view his beloved and much-neglected, oft-maligned Detroit. He asked the big questions and then worked with others to start something small with big implications. Boggs never went to college, but was a prolific writer, thinker, and organizer. He had structural competency in his bones and understood that folks with professional training are at distinct disadvantage inasmuch as their institutional positioning and credentials may block them from immersing themselves in a collective process of struggle and reflection.

Attend carefully to how Boggs focuses on the persistence of exceptionalism as a subtending political myth of the American civic ethos. What political sociologists would call a key or master narrative. According to Boggs, what has the potential to render this exceptionalism less viable and suspect in the eyes of many Americans? The persistence of crises that "wreck other countries." Throughout his five decades of activism, Jimmy Boggs, as he was called by his friends and comrades in Detroit and beyond, lived and witnessed the persistence and deepening of the economic, political, and social crises that have become standard fare in the United States since at least the early 1960s. Such that at the end of his life, he and his comrade and life partner, Grace Lee Boggs, wrote about how the depth and ecological stakes of this crisis changed fundamentally their understanding of the necessity and nature of the social transformations required to address the historical moment: "A revolution is not just for the purpose of correcting past injustices. A revolution involves projecting the notion of a more *human* human being, i.e., a human being who is more advanced in the specific qualities only humans have – creativity, consciousness and self-consciousness, a sense of political and social responsibility" ([6], pp. 15, 19, my emphasis).

Diffusing structural competence into medical education in classroom, clinical, and community spaces means inviting our students into a deeper sense of political and social responsibility as the beginning of a much longer process of individual and collective self-development – the "more human" humanity that Jimmy and Grace Lee Boggs had in mind as they reflected on decades of work. My colleague in Narrative Medicine, Maura Spiegel, in a recent address to an interdisciplinary group of health practitioners, educators, and researchers noted that there is very little space in the professions for true personal development. I suspect one of the reasons for this state of affairs is that the professions are more time-pressed, resources-starved, and bureaucratically encumbered than they were a number of decades ago as the logic of marketization penetrates and colonizes digitally and via other means larger swaths of social life, including those we used to call our private or personal life. Our students would need to question all these dynamics in order to develop a structural literacy regarding their own lives as a critical ethical tool and heuristic of solidarity, while in their training they see constant streams of patients whose illness knots are entangled in the structural forces of stratification and ideological rationalizations of elite power and knowledge.

The late Amiri Baraka, poet, co-founder of the 1960s Black Arts Movement, cultural theorist, and political critic, used to insist during regular public talks in his native Newark, New Jersey, that community educators ground their pedagogy in two fundamental dialectics or mutually inhering apparent opposites that first manifest themselves as intractable contradictions: external limits encircling internal spaces burgeoning with the promise and dynamic potential of self-development and internal limits pressing against collective forward development. Structural competency training implies studying these contradictions in real time and historically and mobilizing one's own self-development as leverage to expand the publicly available spaces and practices for collective development. Part of that is the labors that students can potentially undertake to share widely their respective intellectual and cultural means of production in the service of their patients, the communities they serve, and the ongoing fight for health equity in particular and social justice broadly construed. Our students have a choice to make every day of their lives as professionals and social justice seekers in formation: their human and social capital can be used simply to advance a career path and increase disposable income over a lifetime, and/or it can be redistributed, albeit unevenly, in the struggle to heal, reformat, and even completely restructure our society. These are not minor lessons or political coadjutors to structural competency training and diffusion, but the underlying work of being *more human* by taking on social and political responsibility for breaking internal limits and extending collective external development and vice versa.

The above argument opens up the door to the question of time. Or, to put it more sharply, the times we are traversing and that will shape the rest of our lives no matter what our political affiliations or ideas might be. We are alive at the moment of creation of a palpable and urgent crisis of legitimation and social reproduction in the two national parties that have run the political apparatus of this country since before the Civil War. With the election of Donald Trump, we can discern the advent of a "wrecking" crisis that will bring this nation closer to climate disaster as a way of life and, in the absence of a modicum of the redistribution of economic and symbolic resources, social distension which can potentially spark off open armed conflict that likes of which this nation has not witnessed in living memory. Woe betide those who think that our political and civic institutions are too robust and sedimented to sufferance such a descent into generalized violent social conflict. In short, barring real structural change in our economy and polity, none of these social dynamics will end well. The unique opportunity we have in our classroom, clinical, and community contexts is to make these spaces workshops for another type of future: a laboratory for new, more loving, and radically egalitarian forms of American sociality. To get down to brass tacks: our classrooms can serve our students best by creating spaces of structural competency formation by refusing the temporal logic of the crisis at hand.

In my qualitative methods classroom, slowing down is fostered by the performance of a structured observation. For this exercise, students engage with their privilege and power in the theater of the everyday by slowing down and observing in a location, like a subway stop/car, city steps, or street corner, for 1 h. The goal of the exercise is to get students to reflect on dimensions impacting the chosen setting for the observation-from-a-distance exercise. Students reflect on a variety of aspects of the space like what types of bodies are encouraged or supported by the surroundings and consider the indicators of social/economic/cultural differences and how those indicators relate to each student's personal experience of privilege and power (full list of guiding questions in Appendix 1). This exercise invites students to turn inward and evaluate their own complacency in everyday situations while thinking critically about their role as students and future health professionals within the status quo of structural violence.

Slowing down in this way does not preclude protest, mobilizations, and organizing. Quite the opposite is the case. Rather, slowing down means that we stop responding to the logic of stage-managed urgency and social panic that the enemies of our freedom and liberation in this country expect us to mimic as a way of keeping us off balance and in turmoil. To teach structural competency not as a tool, but as a pedagogy of transformative action is to choreograph with our students and communities of concern a paradoxical double move: as we discern and search for the means of our healing from the structures of violence that delimit our freedom and life chances while in the full confidence that there is nothing wrong with us – not a damn thing wrong with us, but that the system must be transformed root and branch if we are ever going to achieve a full flourishing that many of us call being a human or, to put it more sharply, what freedom might feel like in our bodies/spirits. This work of healing community-building and liberatory activism and organizing requires a slow tempo to counter the commodified and rapid-fire pace of this particular moment of crisis in American racialized capitalism. It also requires collective structures of dialogue and careful discernment of the signs of our times and the seeds of hope contained in the Trumpian disaster on the horizon of our possible futures.

Appendix 1: Structured Observation Guiding Questions

1. What is this space? How does it function? What are its physical characteristics? How is it bounded? How does one gain entry or exit?
2. What are the individual behaviors that are occurring here? What does this space have to do with these behaviors? Are certain behaviors encouraged and others delimited?
3. What are the social interactions that can be observed in this space? How does the setting structure those interactions?
4. Are there odd or outlier activities occurring in this space? Can one observe any patterns or tendencies toward patterns in this setting?
5. Describe the bodies in this space. Does this space change or sustain certain bodily stances or experiences? How does my body feel in this space? How is my subjectivity influenced and influencing the setting under observation?
6. What are the indicators of social/economic/cultural differences that can be observed in this space? How do these indicators relate to my embodiment of social, cultural, and economic privilege and/or inequality and/or difference?

References

1. Ward SM. In love and struggle the revolutionary lives of James and Grace. Chapel Hill: The University of North Carolina Press; 2016.
2. Omi M, Winant H. Racial formation in the United States: from the 1960s to the 1990s. 2nd ed. New York: Routledge; 1994.
3. Dussel E. La Produccion Teorica de Marx: Un Comentario de los Grundrisse. Mexico: Siglo Veinteuno Editores; 1985.
4. Metzl JM, Hansen H. Structural competency: theorizing a new medical engagement with stigma and inequality. Soc Sci Med. 2014;103:126–33.
5. Lorde A. The master's tools will never dismantle the master's house. In: Sister outsider: essays and speeches. New York: Crossing Press; 2007. p. 110–3.
6. Boggs J, Lee Boggs G. Revolution and evolution in the twentieth century. New York: Monthly Review Press; 1974.

Reflections on the Intersection of Student Activism and Structural Competency Training in a New Medical School Curriculum

Cameron Donald, Fabián Fernández, Elaine Hsiang, Omar Mesina, Sarah Rosenwohl-Mack, Aimee Medeiros, and Kelly Ray Knight

The Problem: How Can Student Activists Work with Faculty for Curricular Change

On December 10, 2014, University of California San Francisco (UCSF) medical students staged a die-in to make visible the deaths of Eric Garner,[1] Michael Brown,[2] Alex Nieto,[3] and other victims of police brutality. This action, alongside the collaboration of health professionals and students across the United States inspired a national movement later coined White Coats for Black Lives (WC4BL),[4]

---

[1] Eric Garner (1970–2014) was a husband and father of six children who was choked to death by officers of the New York Police Department. His last words, "I can't breathe," became a rallying cry for the Black Lives Matter Movement (http://www.blackpast.org/aah/garner-eric-1970-2014).

[2] Michael Brown (1996–2014) was a college-bound student shot by an officer of the Ferguson, Missouri Police Department. His body was left out on the street for 4 h. His death became the catalyst for the protests in Ferguson against police brutality.

[3] Alex Nieto (1986–2014) was a full-time scholarship student at Community College of San Francisco earning a criminal justice degree and applying to transfer to a 4-year college program. He was a practicing Buddhist pacifist, a youth mentor, and an active community member. He was shot by four officers of the San Francisco Police Department and inspired the "Frisco 5" Hunger Strike (https://justice4alexnieto.org/).

[4] Members of WC4BL have drafted more of the organization's history in the following article: [1].

C. Donald · F. Fernández · E. Hsiang · O. Mesina · S. Rosenwohl-Mack
University of California, San Francisco, San Francisco, CA, USA

A. Medeiros · K. R. Knight (✉)
Department of Anthropology, History and Social Medicine, University of California, San Francisco, San Francisco, CA, USA
e-mail: kelly.knight@ucsf.edu

© Springer Nature Switzerland AG 2019
H. Hansen, J. M. Metzl (eds.), *Structural Competency in Mental Health and Medicine*,
https://doi.org/10.1007/978-3-030-10525-9_4

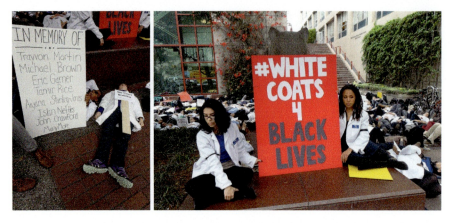

Fig. 1 WC4BL Die-in, Kazandra de la Torre and Kadia Wormley (from left to right). Reprinted with permission from Steve Rhodes: https://www.flickr.com/photos/ari/with/16318354796/

forwarding the notion that "police violence *is* a public health issue."[5] With this foundation set, WC4BL became a national organization of health professionals actively engaging with and dismantling structures that inflict violence on our patients. Since its conception, UCSF's WC4BL chapter has focused on political action and advocacy, community engagement and service, and health professional curricular reform to address local and national manifestations of structural racism and health inequality inside and outside of the classroom and the clinic. One component of this paper synthesizes the perspectives of five UCSF WC4BL members as they reflect on the first year of medical school experience with the new Bridges Curriculum and the impact of advocacy as it connects to the mission of WC4BL (Fig. 1).

During the same period when WC4BL formed as an organization, UCSF medical school was already undergoing a process of curricular reform in undergraduate medical education through the development of the Bridges Curriculum (Bridges). Immediately following the die-in, the UCSF annual retreat scheduled for January 2015 for department chairs and medical education faculty was reorganized to focus on racism and medicine. Two new curricular blocks, Health and the Individual (H&I) and Health and Society (H&S), were developed that increased the curricular time devoted to the social and behavioral sciences through lectures and small groups. One week of the 4-week Health and Individual block dedicated to "Health Disparities," and the two faculty authors (Knight and Medeiros) were junior faculty curricular development committee members focused on content development within that week and its integration with additional content in the H&I and H&S blocks. During the process, students were asked for input and to review proposed content.

---

[5] "Police Violence IS a Public Health Issue" became the rallying cry after UCSF healthcare workers organized to provide medical care to the "Frisco 5" hunger strikes protesting police brutality in San Francisco (http://synapse.ucsf.edu/articles/2016/05/31/urging-police-do-no-harm).

Theoretical Framework

The interventions described here are informed by political movements that attempt to level power inequalities by internally promoting an ethos of coauthorship, and privileging the voices of those with less institutional power, in this case, the students. In keeping with this ethos, this paper was written as a collaboration between two UCSF School of Medicine Department of Anthropology, History, and Social Medicine faculty members and five UCSF WC4BL medical students. These faculty members, intimately involved with the medical school's structural competency content,[6] solicited independent individual reflections from these five students with the suggested prompts: "As I reflect on my first year of medical school, I..." and "UCSF helped students recognize how structural factors influence medicine and health by...." These reflections were then analyzed by the faculty writers, and the reflection's content was categorized by various themes. These themes were presented to and discussed with the students. Themes were updated, content was added, and an organization structure for the piece was proposed. Students then combined portions of their individual narratives into one cohesive piece to capture multiple perspectives with the shared ambition of improving medical education and promoting racial justice. To complement themes that emerged as most salient to the student authors, the two UCSF faculty members (Knight and Medeiros) reflected on the processes that led to the introduction of structural competency into the Bridges Curriculum including lessons learned and recommendations for faculty who would like to attempt similar curricular work at their institutions.

The reflections of the students and faculty members involved in documenting their involvement and/or collaboration with WC4BL and curricular reform raised the following questions:

- What were the medical students' background, experiences, and values before entering their training? How did these sentiments change or evolve throughout the first year?
- How did the background, values, and professional training of the faculty members inform their development of structural competency curriculum?
- How did the students experience the structural competency-related content in the preclinical year? How do their experiences of this content lend to an understanding of structural competency? What were, if any, the successes, highlights, shortcomings, and lessons learned?
- How did faculty initially approach structural competency when introducing the curriculum? What were the key considerations and approaches? What choices were made, and why?
- What were the students' experiences of engaging in dialogue with peers, faculty, and administration around racial justice, health, and structural determinants of health topics?
- How have the faculty members' roles evolved in regard to structural competency since its introduction?

---

[6] Structural competency aims to develop a language and set of interventions to reduce health inequalities at the level of neighborhoods, institutions, and policies. See more at: [2].

The Path

Social Movements and the Field of Medicine
Student Perspectives

Many of the WC4BL members discussed contemporary instances of oppression informing their perspective when they started medical school, as reflected in their narratives of their early involvement with WC4BL:

I began medical school on the sentimental curtails of the June 12, 2016, massacre at the Pulse nightclub where 107 people were either killed or injured by a single armed shooter in this Orlando-based gay club. Though the motives of this attack can never be confirmed, as a queer, black, multiracial man, this moment in history remains searingly salient as an example of the dangerous consequences of homophobia, transphobia, racism, sexism, and toxic nationalism. It continues to tear through my loose notions of safety in the world. Unfortunately, this moment is not unique, and there are reports of violence against people at the margins every day, but this moment in particular is the one I associate with the beginning of my time at UCSF.

I was living in New York City when the #BlackLivesMatter movement began to saturate the media. It was then when I became familiarized with the names of Eric Garner and Michael Brown and truly came into political and social consciousness in a way I had not before, a journey I am still on and continue developing in. During this time, I was working as a care manager in the South Bronx where I had the opportunity of understanding my clients closely – their experiences, goals, and concerns for a system that promised them very little. It was also during this time that our public political discourse was taking a drastic turn and social justice was under attack on many fronts. I took a job at a healthcare think-tank that thought critically about system-level change in delivering healthcare value. I quickly became interested in understanding how this paradigm shift in healthcare delivery was an opportunity for narrowing healthcare disparities, now more than ever, and came into medical school at UCSF acutely attuned to how best develop a skill set that would allow me to address this problem.

Before school, we met online posting about social justice. We met still feeling raw about the summer – the beautiful queer black and brown folks lost under the pulsing lights of the club, the bullets that ripped through Alton Sterling selling bootleg CDs, and all the children who would not be served food by Philando Castile at their local cafeteria.

Faculty Perspectives

The faculty members who worked on the curriculum reform also had significant prior experience addressing structural barriers to health and health care:

Prior to joining the Bridges Curricular committee, I (Knight) had been involved with the Structural Competency Working Group (SCWG),[7] a Bay Area-located collective of physicians, anthropologists, higher education administrators, clergy, and health activists. The SCWG developed a 4-h training that was piloted and evaluated

---

[7] https://www.structcomp.org/

[3]. This training formed the basis of the lecture, "Cultural and Structural Competency," which was first delivered at UCSF in December 2016.

My 20-plus years of experience conducting qualitative health research that focused on drug use/addiction, HIV/AIDS, mental health, reproductive health, and housing instability in US urban poor populations demonstrated the need for a structural analysis in medical education. Many medical students first interact with people who have substance use disorders or people who are experiencing homeless in crisis-driven healthcare situations. The heightened nature of these interactions makes students more likely to endorse exclusively behavioral explanations for poor health and less likely to include structural analyses. They often don't see policies and systems in the patient in front of them. Research on implicit bias also describes stress as contributor to biased assessments and reductionist thinking. The SCWG worked to develop pedagogy that could intervene directly into that interaction and unpack it structurally to address how structures impact health and healthcare. From my perspective this was a critical, yet absent, component of medical education, particularly in the preclinical years.

The call by structural competency developers Metzl and Hansen for a paradigmatic shift in medical education to train future physicians in considering how sociocultural variables – such as race, class, and gender – influence healthcare outcomes resonated with me as an educator and social historian of medicine. I have employed a structural analysis in most of my historical work and have spent the majority of my teaching career educating and collaborating with vulnerable populations in higher education. I felt it was imperative that preclinical medical students better understand how sociopolitical forces including racism, sexism, and homophobia impact patients and healthcare systems and enact humanism in their approach to medicine.

Orientation to Medical School
Student Perspectives

Medical school began at UCSF with the Differences Matter orientation programming, 3 days dedicated to discussing the importance of diversity and manifestations of inequality in the educational environment, workplace, and larger sociopolitical context in which future clinicians would be providing care. During this time, students already began mobilizing around how to affirm their commitment to racial justice.

During orientation week at UCSF, a group of our classmates quickly came together to propose an addendum to our oath for our White Coat Ceremony to stand in solidarity with the recent tragedies faced by countless individuals of color.

It began with a message, "…In light of our nation's ongoing tragedies, I think our White Coat Ceremony could be a powerful opportunity to share our class' solidarity." And within the first week of orientation, we went from four people [on an email] thread to 80 people crowded in [our] medical student lounge trying to come up with a consensus for a statement of solidarity to include in our oath for the ceremony. Ultimately, we could not come to a consensus and ended up laying out flowers on stage, but the Joint Medical Program (JMP) students[8] – in an act of defiance – took an active stand [during the ceremony and, in real-time,] encouraged our class to pledge our work as physicians to fighting issues of poverty, racism, homophobia, and transphobia.

This [attempt at developing a solidarity statement] act drove rifts within our class with a minority of five students in our class vote claiming that these issues had "nothing to do with medicine" and that by focusing on identity politics we were excluding other people who suffer from the narrative.

I think [this student organizing established] an environment of caution within our class regarding when to be defiant and vocal about these systemic injustices.

Students perceived the political and social context at the start of medical school as opening opportunities.

It was hard coming into medical school in the midst of these conflicts, but the bold actions of the Joint Medical Program (JMP) students raised consciousness, drove discussions, and politicized a strong WC4BL community unafraid to take on the administration on issues of racial justice.

The organic way in which this gathering between our classmates occurred quickly made me feel emboldened and humbled to be surrounded by such fiercely determined individuals. The way in which most of my classmates understood issues of racism and economic injustice as the root of many health disparities was inspiring [even though, ultimately], the addendum to the oath was not agreed on by everyone in our class.

Faculty Perspectives

Student activism also encouraged the faculty responsible for curriculum reform to advocate among other faculty for the universal need for attention to health inequalities:

It was heartening to see students create a space for dialogue about social and racial justice during the orientation period. The debates that occurred among the students about the oath ceremony had a parallel on the curriculum committee: there were many discussions about whether or not all medical students needed exposure to structural competency curriculum, as opposed to waiting to introduce such curriculum when students decide to focus on their specific area of practice. The questions among members of the committee were: "Why do dermatologists need to be structurally competent? Why do surgeons?" Part of the development process was to articulate structural competency as a necessary framework for medical education, regardless of a physician's eventual area of practice. It was often necessary in development meetings to clarify that the evidence base on health inequities indicates they occur in all areas of medicines, including dermatology and surgery. There was a need to articulate that having an understanding of the impact of structures on patients' health and healthcare is critical to understanding health. Five decades of

---

[8] The UC Berkeley-UCSF Joint Medical Program (JMP) is a 5-year graduate/medical degree program. Students who are matriculating into the program and attend the same White Coat Ceremony that UCSF medical students attend at the beginning of their first year.

research in health and healthcare disparities were included in the framing of structural competency to underscore this point and connect population-based epidemiological research with clinical care. The social determinants of health were introduced as a launching off point for discussing structural competency.

From Orientation to Medical School
Student Perspectives

After finishing orientation, students were quickly immersed into their core coursework. These students were a part of the newly designed first iteration of the Bridges Curriculum.[9] As part of the Bridges Curriculum, two new content blocks were added to the student's coursework focusing on "Health and the Individual" (H&I) and "Health and Society" (H&S). Much of this course content was grounded in public health and behavioral sciences and social sciences frameworks. It was in these blocks that structural competency content was also introduced as a core principle of medical education and care. Students noted both progress and problems in its implementation.

Many of us in WC4BL were thrilled to learn that the Bridges Curriculum included two blocks devoted to the larger sociopolitical and structural issues that influence our patients' lives and their experiences of medical care. In the winter of our first year, "Health and the Individual" was a 4-week block focusing on health from the perspective of an individual and a family, through social and behavioral sciences. "Health and Society" followed in the spring of that year, as a 4-week block focusing on similar themes but through a societal and structural perspective, and also incorporating health policy and epidemiology. The devotion of 2 full months to the study of the social determinants of health and their surrounding issues in our patients' lives was an exciting development.

The blocks had less work and had open-book exams, and the content is tested on board exams only in the briefest and most cursory way, and, as a consequence, students were less engaged.

In the spring, we had the Health and Society block where we learned about health systems and health insurance and debated our role as physician activists. In discussing these topics with classmates inside and out of the classroom, it became obvious that we all came in with varying levels of comfort and familiarity with the material. Many of us who were perhaps more interested in the material felt it was lacking in academic rigor and was failing to convey the importance of grounding our medical education with these systems in mind.

The Bridges [H&I] Curriculum sparked conversations around the ways that race, ethnicity, LGBTQ identities, addiction, and the physician's role in society were treated in medicine. A lot of the initial lectures laid out terms like "identity" and "culture" through a behavioral psychology lens that felt reductive and oversimplified, losing the interest of students who wanted to study "real medicine" and frustrated students who felt it was not critical enough. Yet later lectures,

---

[9] The UCSF Bridges Curriculum – which launched in August 2016 – is a three-phase, fully integrated curriculum delivered over 4 years (http://meded.ucsf.edu/bridges).

particularly during the H&S block, stimulated conversation in and out of the classroom.

But for the most part, our small group sessions in our Health and the Individual (H&I) and Health and Society (H&S) blocks did not give us the chance to discuss case scenarios through a structural competency lens, instead falling back on discussions of individual factors. While these cases were generally discussed compassionately, conversations often felt incomplete, as they didn't consider the larger picture. I frequently felt frustrated in small groups and in lectures, and many of my classmates made it clear that they would rather be discussing the hard sciences.

The Bridges Curriculum's artificial separation of "Health and the Individual" and "Health and Society" was at times confusing, because the extraction of the individual from society (and vice versa) felt more a practical move to break up the more "clinically and scientifically challenging" blocks of our curriculum than an intentional move based on content. On the other hand, having two entire blocks in the curriculum dedicated to learning about the social determinants of health, as well as having sessions linking the two concepts, was immensely valuable.

WC4BL members also felt frustrated with the way in which course directors responded to student critiques of the block. There were times in which a prioritization of "intellectual discourse" took precedence over acknowledgment of lived experiences.

In the wake of a lecture around reproductive rights that did not present the perspective of the religious right and the student backlash that came with it, the block directors sent out an email pledging to present both sides of an argument. In an era of hyperpolarization, it's important to engage seriously with different perspectives, but it is also important to address and reject ideas assumptions about folks or attempts to silence the lived experience of women, LGBTQ communities, people of color, poor people, and people living with disability. Instead of facilitating frank conversations, our block directors' commitment to "presenting both sides" led to nonsensical all-or-nothing debates around whether physicians should be involved in patient advocacy.

Bridges has done the work of putting issues such as race, class, gender, sexuality, ability, and immigration on the table, but it has done so in silos. Thought-provoking lectures, panels, and patient presentations were coupled with small groups tokenizing its LGBTQ+ and URM [Under-Represented in Medicine] students. Particularly distressing were moments when instructors sent conservative material with "alternative perspectives" after sessions on the ways marginalized people have been harmed by our society or when lectures on race and gender disparities changed direction at the behest of white and male classmates commenting on their "misrepresentation." When members of our class had to then speak up and share the ways they have and continue to survive hate, it became even more difficult to understand why we needed to entertain these requests.

Many individuals in our class witnessed countless instances of classmates feeling uncomfortable with the level of emphasis these blocks placed on discussing issues of race, gender, and privilege. We could see the administration go out of their way to placate their concerns by sending out emails to the entire class explaining the duality of arguments. A small group debate on the importance of advocacy work as physicians presented the urgent need for physician advocacy as a zero-sum game where advocating for patients outside the clinical setting was an "option" in our clinical careers, which left many of us feeling more harm than good was done.

Faculty Perspectives

Faculty members themselves saw the need for additional faculty development to facilitate discussion of challenging topics and for a more holistic approach to in addressing health and healthcare disparities in the curriculum:

Advocating for the inclusion of a structural competency lecture, and additional lectures focused on health and healthcare disparities, was the focus on our efforts on the committee. It was clear after the first year of Bridges that faculty development, training, and capacity were areas that needed further attention, particularly in regard to how to train and support faculty to facilitate difficult conversations that emerge during small groups.

There was a concern that structural competency-related topics would be regulated to either H&I or H&S rather than featured throughout the first 2 years of medical school. A new governance structure was developed to oversee the Bridges Curriculum that included a new committee, Mapping and Integration (M&I), to oversee the longitudinal stewardship and tracking of curriculum topics. Topic Stewards were given the role of overseeing certain topics in the curriculum and reporting to the M&I committee. Emerging topics included gender differences and healthcare disparities. Stewards were encouraged to work with course directors to plan pertinent content, recruit appropriate presenters, develop sessions, and participate in student assessment. This charge gave topic stewards the opportunity to identify gaps in the curriculum both in quantity and quality of related content to their respective topics. Current efforts have identified opportunities for adding more structural competency content and using a structural competency framework when addressing health inequalities.

Deeply Personal
Student Perspectives

The content of H&I and H&S addressed deeply personal topics for many students. How WC4BL members experienced many of their peers' engagement with the material and/or acceptance of their learning generated complicated feelings:

As the blocks (H&I and H&S) unfolded, many of us felt frustrated with their lack of rigor, as well as with the student response to them – many students interpreted these blocks as a time to relax in the midst of an intense curriculum and chose to disengage from the material.

Our reduced workload and focus on critical discussion reawakened unresolved feelings from the White Coat Ceremony. In small groups, we read a case study in which a black woman dating a white man claimed her partner was "not like other white men." A female classmate approached me later to tell me that a man who identifies as white complained about feeling "uncomfortable" and "misrepresented" in the material, rather than fundamentally questioning whether this woman felt unsafe or had experienced issues of intimate partner violence. White students complained privately to other white students they could trust, and without training for facilitators, my friends were often left exhausted from the emotional labor of educating their classmates. An interactive lecture titled "What is Race?" quickly led to questions around why white people weren't allowed to voice their opinions in conversations around race/ethnicity. In this session a person of Jewish descent stated that they felt they could not participate in conversations on race without criticism. Another Chinese-American classmate critiqued affirmative action, opening up about how they felt erased in conversations about race/ethnicity. These sessions opened up a lot of anxieties and questions that are essential in medicine but difficult to navigate early in the curriculum development.

I had a standardized patient give me feedback that asking him his gender was super-fluous because it was obvious. I looked him in the eye and explained, weakly, that while it might be evident to him, it would be a disservice and a violation of trust to make assumptions. I glanced at my team for support, but there wasn't so much as a nod.

It is heartbreaking to hear "the stuff in H&I/H&S is a joke – who cares?" It is heartbreaking to remember Orlando, that when black and brown queer and trans lives were taken, some were misgendered and had their dead names plastered over the internet. That we are advised to put down our signs against police brutality and the prison industrial complex when we enter jails, prisons, and emergency departments as physicians and trainees to work quietly and neatly with law enforcement.

As first-year medical students, we had a panel that made us privy to the "hidden curriculum"[10] of medical school – that on the wards, gathering a social history as stressed by our standardized patient sessions would be the first thing we tossed out of our routine; that our classroom lectures on cultural humility, competency, and respect would be accompanied by in-house patient ridiculing, abject nicknaming, stereotyping, and other forms of inappropriate behaviors by our preceptors, attendings, and PIs; and to succeed during rotations or preceptorships, we would have to swallow the medical hierarchy and socialize to their behaviors, too. We were being given tools we would struggle to use in practice.

Structural Competency
Student Perspectives
WC4BL members highlighted many of the shortcomings of this curricular content but also noted some of its strengths. For some students, the content on structural competency gave students new language, forums, and frameworks to inform their interests in and understandings of the field medicine.

Our lecture in December on cultural and structural competency struck a chord with me, and it gave me a language with which to articulate my frustrations about the way that we as medical students and as people talk about the barriers encountered by those less able to access the resources we enjoy. Cultural competency, though a valuable framework, allows us to minimize the importance of forces that

---

[10] Medical education as is more than simple transmission of knowledge and skills; it is also a socialization process. Wittingly or unwittingly, norms and values transmitted to future physicians often undermine the formal messages of the declared curriculum [4].

shape society – racism, violence, sexism, etc. – by focusing instead on individual factors. But it's not individual factors and individual choices that are the primary drivers of poverty, of the school to prison pipeline, or of racist encounters in a medical setting.

In the healthcare world, structural competency relates closely to public health, as interventions that address the structures that pervade and create society are often found at a policy or systems level; these issues aren't addressed (solely) by training medical professionals to recognize "cultural" differences between groups of people. Our lecture on cultural and structural competency challenged us as students to engage with these sorts of interventions.

In April, another man of color pulled me aside in confidence – as a brilliant science student, he was initially frustrated about how much time we were spending on the social determinants of health. Throughout our small groups, I'd watch him check in and out of conversations or admit that he was more excited to get back to medicine. He confided in me, "I know that all this is important, but I'm still struggling to see what this has to do with medicine – maybe you can help explain it." I tried to talk about white supremacy and how it pervades the logic of medicine – he stared at me distantly. I mentioned the ugly history of "medical apartheid" and how black and brown men, women, and children were denied syphilis treatment in Guatemala[11] and the American South[12]; he remarked that it was a thing of the past. Working with the language of "structural violence," I talked about the way that insurance is structured affects the treatment decisions of our patients [7], and I mentioned how the racialized war on drugs makes physicians less likely to prescribe pain medications to black folks [8] and stressed the ways that the quality of interpreting services impacted patient care [9]. He nodded along and thanked me – he said he was glad to learn more so that he could help his patients. He was as appreciative for this guidance as I was to him when he walked me through cardiac electrophysiology... We were teaching each other through a genuine engagement. Our White Coat Ceremony was validated by the curriculum – these violent structures that we live in had "everything to do with medicine" and were worth learning...

Medicine has never been an exact science. Folks who experience racism, classism, ableism, homophobia, transphobia, Islamophobia, and xenophobia do not get to choose whether these "isms" are a part of their lives or their health. As future medical providers for these individuals, why should we?

The takeaways from the structural competency-based content were in many ways unique for each student and not necessarily in alignment with the "competency" specific framing of the course content. One student argued for a broader justification for education around structural intervention than implied by the term "competency":

---

[11] In Guatemala (1946–1948), the US government infected people with syphilis resulting in at least 83 deaths. In 2010 the United States formally apologized for these experiments. Read More: [5].

[12] In Tuskegee, Alabama (1932–1972), the US government followed the progression of syphilis in 399 black men with 40 wives contracting the disease and 19 children born with congenital syphilis despite the opportunity for treatment. Read More: [6].

I think back on all the times I've been an inadequate advocate for my patients or peers, the times I've struggled to navigate the medical hierarchy. I needed, and still need, guidance. I'd like to think the H&I and H&S blocks would better affirm many of our original motivations to enter medicine if we held ourselves to a higher standard. We need to move beyond the notion of competency, and expand upon what it means to study medicine, become a healer, and galvanize action without turning to trauma porn to justify why we should care.

Faculty Perspectives

In order to make structural competency more legible, the lecture was entitled "Cultural and Structural Competency: Language, Literacy, and Immigration." Cultural competency was a framework that was circulating in the popular vernacular, and some students and many faculty had been exposed to cultural competency. The case example that explored the structural determinants of health developed by Josh Neff in the SCWG built off a real case of a patient affected by policies associated with immigration and impacted by language used to describe his health behaviors and literacy in the SOAP note. Overall, placing structural competency in conversation with familiar constructs helped to situate its importance and avoid critique that it was a "flash-in-the-pan," jargon-y, social science idea.

We had to make some difficult choices when deciding how to pair down the original 4-h training into a 50-min lecture. We developed an Independent Learning Module (ILM) entitled the Social Determinants of Health, to be able to expose the students to that framework, and then very briefly discuss its relationship to structural competency in the lecture. The ILM was a self-guided PowerPoint presentation with voice narration. We also created a reader chapter for the lecture that discussed cultural competency's development and current critiques and the way in which structural competency relates to cultural competency. The ILM and reader chapter freed up time in the lecture to focus on the case example pedagogy and allow for interactive student work, two components of the SCWG 4-h training about which we had received positive feedback.

There was a concern the structural competency lecture was going to be a stand-alone event disparate to other teaching modules addressing social determinants of health that used more traditional methods. We sought out more opportunities to continue the structural competency theme in the preclinical years of instruction, especially during core clerkships, which take place during year two.

The second year of Bridges is referred to as Foundations 2. It is a 14-month program in which students complete their core clinical clerkships, enroll in electives, and attend Foundations Sciences in F2 day (FS-in-F2 Days) 1 day every other week. Each day has a topic, such as genetics, cancer, and addiction. During the development of the FS-in-F2 day calendar, we proposed a day dedicated to the foundational science of structural competency, and it was accepted.

The curriculum development team for this day comprised of volunteers from an action group dedicated to promoting the most inclusive learning environment in the school of medicine. This group was part of a larger initiative (Differences Matter[13]) that grew out of the School of Medicine's response to the 2014 die-in discussed in the introduction to this essay. The result of our effort was a 6-h long day of instruction on the foundational science of structural competency. Teaching modules included a critical look at evidence-based medicine, a presentation on the impact of racism in gynecology, a training session on strategies for promoting health from a population-level to the individual, and a roundtable discussion by physicians on how structural competency language can promote better health outcomes for vulnerable populations.

The FS-in-F2 day in Structural Competency also gave us the opportunity to champion more systemic changes to the curriculum. As each foundational science day was to adhere to at least one of the 12 "FS Principles,"[14] we suggested an additional principle – Social Medicine. We defined social medicine as "the study of how political, economic, and social structures – and their resulting conditions – impact health, disease, and the practice of medicine." Our intent was to encourage the integration of structural competency-related content and analyses to FS-in-F2 curriculum as a whole and to consider social medicine as a foundational science on par with existing principles, such as immunology and genetics.

Addressing Shortcomings
Student Perspectives
In light of the many shortcomings these students were experiencing, many found support and solace in the UCSF WC4BL chapter and utilized this space to address the aforementioned issues. The ways in which these members addressed the problems they were recognizing were varied and in many ways very impactful. Students were also cognizant of their own limitations in regard to addressing these issues.

The understatement of the year would be to simply express an appreciation for the Bridges Curriculum. It is a beautiful thing to spend weeks at a time studying the open secrets of racism and other structural barriers in medicine. But it has been during White Coats for Black Lives gatherings where I found solidarity and strength in being able to say: this is not enough.

We talked in WC4BL meetings about the often-lackluster student response to the blocks and about our personal frustrations hearing our friends and classmates speak dismissively about the content or the time devoted to it. Even some classmates who appreciated the importance of the content felt that we spent too much time on it, saying that the curriculum should not have devoted the same amount of time to the H&S block as it did to the cardiology block. As frustrating as it is to feel that assessment drives engagement, we talked in WC4BL about how critical reflection pieces or even a separate individual project might be useful and/or necessary drivers of more robust student engagement in those blocks.

---

[13] https://differencesmatter.ucsf.edu/

[14] Twelve FS Principles: anatomy, behavioral sciences, siostatistics and epidemology, microbiology, pathology, pharmacology, physiology, aging, immunology, molecular and cell biology, nutrition, and genetics

In early winter my classmates in WC4BL came together to think critically about how to best push the administration to advance many of the topics we were covering in our curriculum. We divided into three pillars to conduct sexual education workshops with black elders in the Bayview community, work closely with the administration involved in curriculum development to define anti-racism competencies, and collaborate with the national WC4BL chapter to develop our Racial Justice Report Card that graded the UCSF community on issues of institutional diversity and preclinical education, among others. Our chapter members worked tirelessly to research and develop the document and present it to our classmates and the UCSF community at large. My experience working on the Report Card with my classmates was inspiring. I learned about the "Basement People,"[15] medical apartheid,[16] history of labor unions, and worker rights[17] and began to contextualize my training as a medical student and how it has come to be what it is today largely on the backs of people of color. I struggled to reason why these historical perspectives were not taught to us during our preclinical curriculum. We are now working with the Differences Matter curriculum development committee to integrate this content for the future. Our Report Card brought attention to the clinical encounters we are exposed to and how they are limited in the diversity of clinical experiences. Our recommendations were heard, and we will now be having clinical encounters involving limited-English proficiency patients to understand how to navigate translation services. The work WC4BL has done has created modes of institutional accountability in ways that we did not expect. We are grateful for the administration's commitment to work collaboratively with us. Our continual engagement with our classmates and the UCSF community at large, as well as the efforts being made to refine our curriculum to better introduce and teach structural competency to future classes, will surely enlighten our classmates to understand and participate in dismantling the structures that are preventing our patients from the best possible care.

Despite these successes, we know there is more work to be done. This includes the incorporation of content from H&I and H&S into other preclinical blocks and into the inquiry curriculum,[18] rather than allowing the content to be siloed into those two units. Better training of small group facilitators on topics of race and racism is another critical next step. The curriculum should specifically include structural violence education and anti-racism training. Additionally, community members ought to be invited not only to speak during the H&I and H&S blocks but also to have a role in structuring and/or facilitating sessions in these blocks.

---

[15] In 1968, UCSF facilities were segregated, and people of color had to go to the basement to eat or use the bathroom. The "basement people," as they were called, organized a meeting in Cole Hall that led to the birth of the Black Caucus and a transformation of the UCSF campus (https://www.ucsf.edu/news/2013/05/105576/beloved-ucsf-professor-dan-lowenstein-delivers-inspirational-last-lecture).

[16] Read More: [10].

[17] Read More: [11].

[18] The inquiry curriculum is a longitudinal component of Bridges that engages students in research appraisal and the generation of new knowledge (http://meded.ucsf.edu/bridges/inquiry-curriculum).

The efforts of WC4BL [over the school year] were expansive, spanning from local and national advocacy efforts, to curricular development and community outreach... Much of this of work was imperfect, human. It required limitless effort from limited bodies. As such, most of these efforts were met with critique, and the critiques were usually met with surprising grace. Pursuing a just world is an iterative and tiring process. By the end of the year, I felt tired but also empowered by the fact that UCSF is an institution so committed to modeling what equitable, ethical medicine can be. Having these values myself, and seeing these values reflected in both an institution I am a part of, and among peers and mentors I am surrounded by, inform and motivate the work I will continue to pursue.

Key Learnings

We, as faculty interested in and advocating for structural competency instruction throughout the 4-year Bridges Curriculum, are grateful for the courageous actions taken by medical students in providing candid feedback and suggesting changes to the curriculum that will better prepare them as future physicians and promote health and social justice. As a result of their efforts, student input helped shape milestones which inform the seven guiding competencies of the medical school curriculum. These changes include explicit language about the role of race, class, and gender in clinical care. The UCSF WC4BL Racial Justice Report Card offered suggestions to extend the structural competency-related content in the first year and provided specific, critical feedback for the revision of the introduction to structural competency lecture that has been incorporated. These students are also playing a vital role in the shaping of year two curriculum as several WC4BL members now serve on a design team for structural competency curriculum development. As the Bridges Curriculum evolves, administrators have championed the continued input from these students and have made changes accordingly.

Students' reflective conclusions were as follows:

We acknowledge that the relative success of our institutional advocacy efforts have largely been due to UCSF's receptive institutional climate. Far too often, healthcare systems, and medical educators, and administrators are overly cautious or even antagonistic toward issues of racial justice. Yet the receptive support of WC4BL, espoused by various administrators at UCSF, sets the tone for a different type of relationship. A few days after the Pulse Shooting in Orlando, Vice Dean of Education at UCSF Dr. Catherine Lucey sent an email to the medical community lamenting the violence asking: "What can we, as professionals committed to saving lives and alleviating suffering, do? How can we help to make this madness stop? It is far too easy to say that it is far too hard a problem to tackle. While I don't have the answer, I believe that collectively we must commit to taking steps small and large to prevent these events from recurring." During our orientation, Dean Lucey called combating racism the "AIDS epidemic of our time," challenging us as medical students to fight against it. With administrative support, WC4BL was able to organize in the Multicultural Resource Center and get reimbursed for food and materials. We were able to reach out to administrators and get support writing our Racial Justice Report Card. While our chapter recognizes a diversity of tactics, we were fortunate enough to have a good working relationship with the administration, driving change from without and within.

Finally, while our attempts to work with the UCSF administration to improve the School of Medicine's curriculum redefine safe, inclusive pedagogical methods and learning environments and inspire public discourse on issues of social injustice were met with unwavering support, we want to recognize that there are limits to institutional work. As a part of the new curriculum, H&I and H&S promised to train us how to navigate issues of identity, structural violence, and power differentials between patients and providers. Yet the inherent context of this curriculum often lent itself to overly academic and/or poorly facilitated conversations, existing merely as intellectual debates. Additionally, this pedagogical structure can and does exhaust students of color. It is these students who are left burdened with the task of educating their classmates through the vulnerable process of exposing their own life experiences. Idiosyncratically, the aforementioned context forced many of us to stress the importance of this curriculum despite the fact that we personally were not engaging at the level we had hoped because of this fatigue. As such, we believe that understanding many of these concepts requires leaving the confines of the classroom. Throughout the school year, WC4BL and the Multicultural Resource Center became a safe haven where we could voice our frustrations, discuss issues with the curriculum, and envision a different medical school experience. It was in these meetings that we felt most comfortable when engaging with these challenging concepts, affirmed each other's experiences, and began expanding our efforts to the larger Bay Area and national community. Ultimately, it was this space that allowed us to dream beyond. While we can continue to make our curriculum more radical and inclusive, there will always be a need for spaces beyond the confines of the institution where we can socialize, organize, and dream in community.

References

1. Charles D, et al. White coats for black lives: medical students responding to racism and police brutality. J Urban Health. 2015;92(6):1007–10.
2. Metzl JM, Hansen H. Structural competency: theorizing a new medical engagement with stigma and inequality. Soc Sci Med. 2014;103:126–33.
3. Neff J, Knight KR, Satterwhite S, Nelson N, Matthews J, Holmes SM. Teaching structure: a qualitative evaluation of a structural competency training for resident physicians. J Gen Intern Med. 2016;32(4):430–3.
4. Mahood SC. Medical education. Can Fam Physician. 2011;57(9):983–5.
5. Rodriguez MA, García R. First, do no harm: the US sexually transmitted disease experiments in Guatemala. Am J Public Health. 2013;103(12):2122–6.
6. Gamble VN. Under the shadow of Tuskegee: African Americans and health care. Am J Public Health. 1997;87(11):1773–8.
7. Hadley J. Sicker and poorer – the consequences of being uninsured: a review of the research on the relationship between health insurance, medical care use, health, work, and income. Med Care Res Rev. 2003;60(2_suppl):3S–75S.
8. Pletcher MJ, et al. Trends in opioid prescribing by race/ethnicity for patients seeking care in US emergency departments. JAMA. 2008;299(1):70–8.

9. Pérez-Stable EJ, Napoles-Springer A, Miramontes JM. The effects of ethnicity and language on medical outcomes of patients with hypertension or diabetes. Med Care. 1997;35(12):1212–9.

10. Washington HA. Medical apartheid: the dark history of medical experimentation on Black Americans from colonial times to the present. New York: Doubleday Books; 2006.

11. Becker ER, Sloan FA, Steinwald B. Union activity in hospitals: past, present, and future. Health Care Financ Rev. 1982;3(4):1.

The Structural Competency Working Group: Lessons from Iterative, Interdisciplinary Development of a Structural Competency Training Module

Joshua Neff, Seth M. Holmes, Shirley Strong, Gregory Chin, Jorge De Avila, Sam Dubal, Laura G. Duncan, Jodi Halpern, Michael Harvey, Kelly Ray Knight, Elaine Lemay, Brett Lewis, Jenifer Matthews, Nick Nelson, Shannon Satterwhite, Ariana Thompson-Lastad, and Lily Walkover

No one has a right to work with poor people unless they have a real analysis of why people are poor.
(Barbara Major, The People's Institute for Survival and Beyond, New Orleans [1])

Building Social Analysis into Curricula for Health Professionals

Structural competency incorporates frameworks from the social sciences into clinical training. This is done in hopes of preparing clinicians to recognize and respond to the connections between social, political, and economic structures and their

J. Neff (✉) · J. Halpern
UC Berkeley-UCSF Joint Medical Program, Berkeley, CA, USA
e-mail: jhalpern@berkeley.edu

S. M. Holmes
Division of Society and Environment, Joint Program in Medical Anthropology, Berkeley
Center for Social Medicine, University of California, Berkeley, Berkeley, CA, USA
e-mail: sethmholmes@berkeley.edu

S. Strong · E. Lemay
Samuel Merritt University, Oakland, CA, USA
e-mail: sstrong@samuelmerritt.edu; ELemay@samuelmerritt.edu

© Springer Nature Switzerland AG 2019   53
H. Hansen, J. M. Metzl (eds.), *Structural Competency in Mental Health and Medicine*,
https://doi.org/10.1007/978-3-030-10525-9_5

G. Chin
Department of Neurological Surgery, University of California, San Francisco,
San Francisco, CA, USA

J. De Avila
University of Chicago Pritzker School of Medicine, Chicago, IL, USA

S. Dubal
Department of Medical Anthropology, University of California, Berkeley, Berkeley, CA, USA

University of California, San Francisco, San Francisco, CA, USA

L. G. Duncan · S. Satterwhite
Medical Scientist Training Program, Department of Anthropology, History and Social
Medicine, University of California, San Francisco, San Francisco, CA, USA
e-mail: shannon.Satterwhite@ucsf.edu

K. R. Knight
Department of Anthropology, History and Social Medicine, University of California,
San Francisco, San Francisco, CA, USA
e-mail: kelly.knight@ucsf.edu

M. Harvey
San Jose State University, San Jose, CA, USA
e-mail: michael.harvey@sjsu.edu

B. Lewis
Oregon Health Sciences University, Portland, OR, USA
e-mail: lewibr@ohsu.edu

J. Matthews
Department of Adolescent Medicine, University of California San Francisco Benioff
Children's Hospital Oakland, Oakland, CA, USA

N. Nelson
Internal Medicine Residency Program, Highland Hospital, Oakland, CA, USA

University of California, San Francisco, San Francisco, CA, USA
e-mail: nnelson@alamedahealthsystem.org

A. Thompson-Lastad
Osher Center for Integrative Medicine, University of California, San Francisco, San
Francisco, CA, USA
e-mail: Ariana.Thompson-Lastad@ucsf.edu

L. Walkover
Global Health, Drexel University, Philadelphia, PA, USA

downstream effects on health and healthcare. To paraphrase the words of Barbara Major above, these frameworks can help providers develop a real analysis of the *social structures* (see definition) that make certain people poor – and thereby also more vulnerable to preventable disease, injury, and death. Similarly, social science frameworks can enable providers to recognize the structural influences on the organization and practice of healthcare. In other words, social science frameworks can help healthcare providers attend and respond to the influence of structures both within and beyond formal clinical roles.

> **Definition: Social Structures**
> The policies, economic systems, and other institutions (judicial system, schools, etc.) that have produced and maintain modern social inequities as well as health disparities, often along the lines of social categories such as race, class, gender, and sexuality

There remains much to learn, however, about how to introduce social science analysis into the training of healthcare professionals. Active questions include:

- *Who should be trained in the social analysis underpinning structural competency?* Which professionals and at which stage of their training or careers? Who tends to be most or least receptive?
- *How should such social analysis be taught?* By whom and through which pedagogic techniques? How much curricular time is necessary to make a meaningful and lasting contribution to participants' thinking and practice?
- *What content should be included?* Of the wide array of social science literature and other relevant content available, what should be emphasized within structural competency?

Since 2014, the Structural Competency Working Group (SCWG) – an interdisciplinary group of healthcare providers, scholars, students, and community health advocates based in the San Francisco Bay Area – has been exploring the above questions by designing, implementing, and evaluating classroom-based structural competency training modules for healthcare professionals. At the time of writing this, training had been implemented over 35 times – in a range of formats and for providers in a range of health-related disciplines (Table 1).

This chapter describes the SCWG, which includes many of the authors of this chapter, and our process through the development, refinement, adaptation, and dissemination of our structural competency training. We also share lessons learned thus far from our efforts to operationalize structural competency training for healthcare professionals. These include the value of practicing "impractical" thinking; the importance of iterative, interdisciplinary collaboration; the necessity to make

Table 1 SCWG structural competency training sites[a]

Alameda Health System (Highland Hospital) Internal Medicine Residency (3x)
Contra Costa Family Medicine Residency
HEART-IM Clerkship – University of New Mexico School of Medicine (2x)
MiMentor (pre-health undergraduates)
Oregon Health Sciences University (4x)
Prep Medico (pre-health undergraduates)
Samuel Merritt University School of Nursing (2x)
Santa Rosa Family Medicine Residency
Society for Teachers of Family Medicine
UC Berkeley School of Public Health (2x)
UC Berkeley-UCSF Joint Medical Program (4x)
UCSF Benioff Children's Hospital Oakland – pediatric residents
UCSF Benioff Children's Hospital Oakland – social work trainees (3x)
UCSF Department of Physical Therapy and Rehabilitation Science
UCSF Global Health Master's Program
UCSF HEAL Initiative Global Health Fellowship (4x)
UCSF Internal Medicine Residency Primary Care Program at San Francisco General Hospital (SFPC)
UCSF School of Medicine – 1st year students (3x)
UCSF School of Nursing – Masters Entry Program in Nursing (nurse practitioner) students

[a]As of writing in summer 2018

content "sticky" and balance pedagogic approaches; the benefits of feedback-driven pedagogic development; and strategies for adapting and disseminating structural competency for diverse audiences.

Theoretical Framework: Practicing "Impractical" Thinking

The SCWG grew out of an initiative called Envisioning Radical Experiments in Clinical Medicine, or "Rad Med." Rad Med originally consisted of two working groups: one focused on medical education and the other focused on the intersection of mental health, policing, and incarceration. Rad Med's medical education group, which evolved into the Structural Competency Working Group, aimed to introduce social science-informed critical perspectives into medical education and clinical practice. Meeting for two hours every other week, we started by reading and discussing relevant articles and book chapters – e.g., Geiger [2], Holmes and Ponte [3], Metzl and Hansen [4], Pine [5], and Rivkin-Fish [6]. Through these readings and discussions, we settled on structural competency as a useful guiding framework for our efforts.

Over our first semester, MD/anthropology PhD student Sam Dubal introduced a number of imaginative proposals designed to push clinical practice to confront unjust social, political, and economic structures. For instance, he created sample "radical" medical histories incorporating structural and symbolic factors that lead to sickness, as well as corresponding structural "prescriptions" that could be offered by clinicians in a structurally responsive medicine. Such creative exercises helped us establish, as a core orientation for our group and our training efforts, a commitment to giving ourselves and others permission to think, as physician-anthropologist Seth Holmes put it, "impractically" as well as "practically" when considering interventions in medical training and practice. Our goal in highlighting that which at first appears impractical was to avoid constraining our imaginations with received notions of what is possible – which we felt could lead us to set our sights too low and stifle "out-of-the-box" thinking. We hoped to shake some of our inurement to the status quo by keeping in view our most ambitious hopes for medical practice and training – and for society at large.

As the semester continued, we decided to focus on developing our first structural competency training. Seth Holmes and MD/MS student Josh Neff began discussions with a family medicine residency program about conducting this session with their residents. Ultimately, we arranged to run a three hour training for their cohort of interns, at the end of their first year of residency, in June 2015. We decided also to prepare a similar training for the program's core faculty, informed by literature suggesting that faculty who receive ongoing education in parallel to their trainees can better reinforce (rather than contradict) trainees' learning [7–10].

The Path: Iterative, Interdisciplinary Collaboration

With our pilot training approaching in early summer, our group worked steadily through winter and spring 2015 to develop a classroom-based structural competency training module that would be relevant, compelling, and impactful for family medicine residents and faculty.

During our twice-monthly meetings, we brainstormed what to include in the training. Informed by these discussions, in the weeks between meetings, Josh Neff – whose medical anthropology master's project focused on the development, implementation, and evaluation of this training – worked to generate training materials. At the following meeting, Josh would present to the group what he had developed; based on this, the group offered feedback and brainstormed next steps, which would once again guide Josh's efforts until the next meeting. Group members' diverse experience was essential to this process. Having clinicians, social science scholars, administrators, activists, students, and patients collaborating together – in real-time, in person – yielded ideas and approaches for training that we otherwise could never have developed. This interdisciplinary group composition, enabled in part by members' involvement in various academic settings, was cultivated by proactively striving to broaden the variety of backgrounds and perspectives of those involved in the group.

Week by week, piece by piece, the training took shape. We decided to organize the training into three main sections:

1. How structures affect patient health
2. How structures affect the practice of healthcare
3. Strategies for responding to structures in and beyond the clinic

In all three sections, we planned to emphasize the importance of *structural humility* (see definition). The content of the training and key aspects of our process are described in the following section.

Definition: Structural Humility
Coined by Metzl and Hansen [4], structural humility highlights the importance of respecting and deferring to the knowledge of patients and communities, rather than only or primarily considering the knowledge of the health "expert." It also encourages clinicians to follow the lead of patients and communities in developing appropriate, sustainable interventions to address harmful social structures.

Developing the Training: Making Content "Sticky" and Balancing Pedagogic Approaches

As we developed the various components of the training, we were guided by a few core intentions. First, we did not only want to interest or persuade participants – we wanted the core themes of our training to stay with them long afterward. As some of us came to say, we wanted to make sure that the training was "sticky." We pushed ourselves to think creatively about how we could present the material to facilitate this. In support of this effort, we also wanted to make sure the various components of training were clear and cohesive, with key themes reiterated throughout the session. And we knew it would be important to strike a balance between reflection, discussion, and didactics. Too much time spent on didactics and learners would not have a chance to process and integrate the material, and their attention would wane. Conversely, a brief session with no didactics at all would be unlikely to offer novel frameworks and perspectives.

Early in our process of creating the training, we wrestled with how we could succinctly and memorably illustrate the concept of social structures (definition above) and the impact of structures on patient health. These conversations prompted Josh Neff to develop a diagram – revealed incrementally in an animated slide – that illustrates how one patient's life course and health are influenced by large-scale social, political, and economic structures (Fig. 1). These simple animated diagrams, which

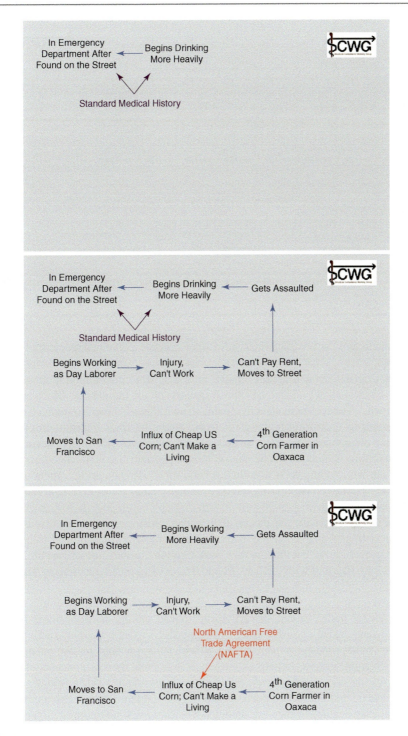

Fig. 1 Patient arrow diagram

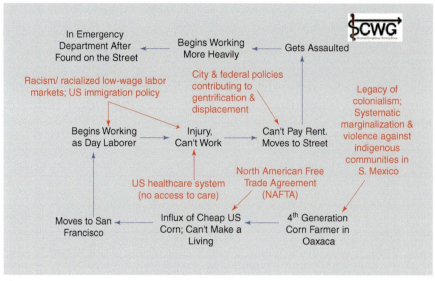

Fig. 1 (continued)

we came to call "arrow diagrams," have since become a core pedagogic tool of our trainings.

This original arrow diagram – based on a case from the ethnographic work of James Quesada [11] – sketches the trajectory of an indigenous Mexican corn farmer who is unable to make a living due to an influx of cheap American corn. He immigrates to California looking for work, where he finds intermittent employment as a day laborer. However, he gets injured on the job. This injury prevents him from working, which means he can no longer pay rent. He starts sleeping on the street and while doing so is assaulted several times. This ongoing trauma triggers increased alcohol consumption, which eventually leads to his arrival in the emergency room.

The slides start with the pieces of this man's history most often discussed in clinical settings – that he needed medical care after losing consciousness secondary to heavy alcohol use. Facilitators then walk through the above-described life course step-by-step, starting with his background as a corn farmer. After tracing his story, structures that likely influenced his trajectory are shown in red.

Based on this slide, internal medicine physician Nick Nelson wrote up a sample chart note for such a patient for participants to read and discuss prior to our sharing this slide and the patient's trajectory (see Appendix A). Our hope in this activity was to interest and prime participants to engage with the arrow diagram. We intended the arrow diagram, in turn, to help us introduce and define the key concepts of *structural violence* and *structural vulnerability* (see definitions) [12–15]. In order to balance didactic and interactive portions and to give residents a chance to apply these concepts, we decided to then ask them to share examples of structural violence and structural vulnerability they had witnessed, in the clinic or otherwise.

Definition: Structural Violence
"Structural violence is one way of describing social arrangements that put individuals and populations in harm's way... The arrangements are structural because they are embedded in the political and economic organization of our social world; they are violent because they cause injury to people" – *Farmer* et al [12].

Definition: Structural Vulnerability
The risk that an individual experiences as a result of structural violence – including their location in multiple socioeconomic hierarchies. Structural vulnerability is not caused by, nor can it be repaired solely by, individual agency or behaviors.

In addition to discussing the ways in which structures affect health, we felt it essential to highlight how structural influences are often overlooked. Specifically, we wanted to offer participants language for discussing ideology, internalized and often implicit, that can habituate us to look for individual and "cultural" level explanations for poor health outcomes – often overlooking the structural determinants of harm in the process. We decided to introduce this concept in terms of "naturalizing inequality" (see definition) [13, 16–18]. Again we planned time for residents to reflect on and share how they had observed inequality being naturalized in their clinical and personal experience.

Definition: Naturalizing Inequality
When inequality and structural violence are justified by, or go unacknowledged due to, nonstructural explanations for structurally mediated harms/inequities. These nonstructural explanations – which often emphasize individual behaviors, "cultural" characteristics, or biologized racial categories – help preserve social inequities by giving the impression that the status quo is "natural," in the sense of not being primarily social or structural in origin.

Table 2 Structural competency training learning objectives	1. Identify the influences of structures on patient health
	2. Identify the influences of structures on the practice of healthcare
	3. Generate strategies to respond to the influences of structures in the clinic
	4. Generate strategies to respond to structural influences beyond the clinic
	5. Describe structural humility as an approach to apply in and beyond the clinic

We set aside the last portion of section 1 to define structural competency, including a discussion of our learning objectives for the session as a whole (Table 2). We also here planned to discuss briefly the relationships between structural competency and the frameworks of cultural competency and the social determinants of health (SDOH). Our key point with respect to cultural competency was that cultural frameworks – while potentially helpful in training providers to provide care cross-culturally – are not well suited to analyzing health disparities that have primarily structural rather than cultural origins [4, 19, 20]. As for SDOH compared to structural competency, we first of all noted that SDOH is a broad umbrella that sometimes includes a structural analysis – including in the work of those who framed the term [21–23]. We observed, however, that curricula framed in terms of the SDOH sometimes fail to mention the various structural factors that create and maintain inequities – even as they describe the epidemiology connecting social inequity and health outcomes (Fig. 2). As a result, these curricula can inadvertently naturalize inequalities, and they generally do not discuss strategies for intervening on the structural drivers of inequalities [24–26]. To highlight this distinction, we started introducing a phrase Josh Neff had said at a meeting: "the structural determinants of the social determinants of health."

In the second section of the training, we sought to cultivate awareness of the structures that affect the practice of healthcare. We decided to minimize didactics in this section, instead giving participants an opportunity to reflect upon the social, political, and economic structures that they had experienced as enabling or impeding their delivery of care. We also invited the participants to apply the concepts of structural violence and naturalizing inequality to their and their colleagues' practice and trajectories – with particular attention to realities such as the stress and burnout experienced by providers due to their participation in structures of violence.

The third and final section focused on strategies for responding to structures in and beyond the clinic. Guided by our commitment to practice "impractical" thinking, we asked participants to imagine, share, and discuss both "practical" and "impractical" strategies for addressing harmful structural influences on health and healthcare. Again we felt that participants would be best served by a reflection and

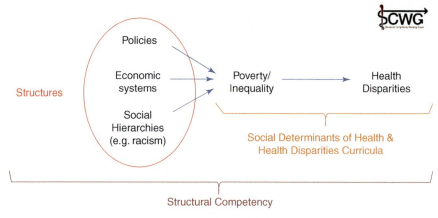

Fig. 2 Structural competency and SDOH curricula

discussion-driven approach, as this would allow them to brainstorm strategies relevant to their particular practice settings and circumstances.

Inspired in part by our literature review of related trainings, we recognized that if discussions about structural and other societal issues focus too heavily on describing problems and too little on ways to address them, participants would be more likely to feel discouraged and disempowered [27–29]. With this in mind, we decided to close the training on a hopeful note, emphasizing the possibility of structural change through collective work – including the California Nursing Association's successful campaign to cap nursing ratios in California, which has been shown to benefit patients as well as nurses [30, 31].

With the resident training thus laid out, our last step was to prepare a shorter version of the training for faculty, who had only two hours available. We wanted to make sure that the faculty were familiar with the range of material we covered with residents, so we shortened the training's interactive portions.

Implementation and Evaluation: Identifying Strengths and Weaknesses

The resident and faculty training were implemented in June 2015. We felt these went smoothly, and residents and faculty appeared to be engaged throughout their respective sessions. In post-training written-response surveys, both residents and faculty provided predominantly positive feedback – some emphatically so – along with a number of critiques and helpful suggestions for how the training could be improved. For a sample of residents' responses, see our article in the Journal of General Internal Medicine in 2017 [32].

Following these sessions, Josh Neff analyzed participant surveys and conducted a focus group with residents one month post-training, to learn more about their perspectives after they had returned to clinic and to find out how "sticky" the training had in fact been. Our expectation in anticipation of this focus group was that the residents would still generally feel positively about the session. However, we also expected that, with the passage of a month's time and the many demands of residency, our session would have faded from the forefront of their minds.

To our surprise, we found that, to the contrary, the training was still very much on residents' minds. The residents in attendance – all those not on call or on vacation – highlighted that they were "thinking about it constantly." Some said this awareness was influencing how they related to patients – as one resident put it, "It has been very effective in helping to build a partnership with patients." They also commented that having a "shared vocabulary" with one another made it "a lot easier to talk about" structural influences on health.

Many residents, however, also reported that their heightened awareness of the structural influences on health was leading to a sense of distress. They said that the extent and seeming immutability of this influence was discouraging when they encountered structures harming their patients' lives. This sentiment was particularly acute, they reported, because they already felt overwhelmed by how little time they had with patients and how much medicine they still needed to learn. Despite this experience, they advocated unanimously for the expansion of structural competency training. Again, see Neff et al. for resident quotes and further discussion of the evaluation of our pilot effort [32].

Three specific suggestions for future structural competency education efforts emerged from this conversation. First, the residents recommended providing more examples of how healthcare providers have responded to structural issues. They appreciated space and time to brainstorm responses, but they wanted to hear more about past and current efforts to address harmful structures and work toward positive social change. Second, they recommended including structural competency during earlier stages of training, before trainees are expected to efficiently manage the many demands of providing patient care. As one resident put it, "It would be good to develop tools before… you need them in 10 minutes." Third, they recommended expanding structural competency training into a more in-depth, longitudinal curriculum.

From Key Learnings to Revisions: Feedback-Driven Pedagogic Development

Based on evaluations and our observations from our pilot effort, in the fall of 2015, we worked to improve the training. First and foremost, we wanted to address the extent of the distress described by residents. We felt that incorporating more examples of providers' responses to harmful structures, as suggested by the residents, would be necessary toward this end. We thought, however, that this might not be sufficient – that it would be important also to normalize a range of possible responses, recognizing that many feel some level of distress when reflecting on injustice – and that this is a potentially appropriate response. Additionally, we suspected that some of the discomfort experienced by residents was related to the fact that people who choose to go into clinical healthcare frequently have action and outcome-oriented dispositions (several authors included). There is a tendency for providers to want, and perhaps to some extent expect, to be able to fix problems. This orientation can make it uncomfortable to discuss challenges – such as trying to change unjust social structures – that cannot be addressed primarily through individual effort or on a predictable timeframe.

We also felt it important to develop further the second section of the training, which addresses the structural influences on the practice of healthcare. First, we noticed that this section was not much emphasized by participants in our evaluations, which led us to believe there was room to make this section "stickier." Second, we thought it important to enhance this section to the extent that residents' distress was connected to structural factors influencing their delivery of care – for instance, the fact that they felt they already had too much to do in too little time. Though we did not believe that a greater focus on the structural influences on healthcare practice would alleviate distress in and of itself, we felt it important for them to keep in view the structural determinants of these experiences of distress and overwhelm.

In response to the residents' experience and suggestions, we created several new components of section 3. First, led by pediatrician Jen Matthews, anthropologist Kelly Knight, MD/anthropology PhD students Shannon Satterwhite and Laura G. Duncan, and Josh Neff, we developed the "levels of intervention" activity, to help trainees recognize the different levels of potential engagement (Table 3). In this activity, participants are divided into groups, and each group is asked to brainstorm possible responses to structural violence at a particular level. Groups then share what they considered, and we lead a discussion of the interconnections of the levels as well as the possibility of engaging in different levels over time. Prior evaluations had suggested that some participants had concluded that structural competency implies they should become directly involved in policy-level work; we hoped that this exercise would help address participant distress by making clear our view that there are various scales at which providers can beneficially act based on their recognition of the harms caused by large-scale structures.

Also in response to trainee distress in the first iterations, we prepared a range of examples of provider responses to structural issues at various levels, both historical and contemporary. The examples ranged from historical examples such as the Black Panther Party's People's Free Health Clinics and the Delta Health Center in Mississippi – and the legacies of each – to more recent examples including ACT-UP's housing activism for AIDS patients and the California Nurses Association's influence on state healthcare policy [2, 30, 33, 34].

We closed section 3 of the training with Shirley Strong, Chief Diversity Officer at Samuel Merritt University, presenting her definition of the "Beloved Community" (see definition). In our group meetings, Shirley had discussed the concept of Beloved Community, as articulated by Martin Luther King, Jr., as a guiding principle in her career as an advocate and activist. She noted that people trying to address harmful social structures too frequently offer critique without articulating a positive vision. Beloved Community is Shirley's guiding principle for developing such a vision.

> **Shirley Strong's Definition of Beloved Community**
> An inclusive, interconnected consciousness – based on love, justice, compassion, responsibility, shared power, and a deep respect for all people, places, and things – that radically transforms individuals and restructures institutions

We made just one major change to section 2: adding the "provider arrow diagram" (Fig. 3). This diagram returns to the case presented at the start of section 1, focusing this time on the structural influences behind the provider's trajectory over time. It follows the provider as they slide from idealism toward cynicism over their

Table 3 Levels of intervention

Levels of intervention		Example(s)
1.	Individual	Develop awareness of and work to counter one's own implicit racism/bias
2.	Interpersonal	Apply structural thinking to approach patients without blame or judgment
3.	Clinic/ institutional	Diversify staff and provide structural competency training to all staff
4.	Community	Collaborate with community members/organizations to do community organizing around affordable housing for vulnerable patients
5.	Policy	Participate in collective efforts to establish universal healthcare, reform immigration laws/practices that harm one's patients, etc.
6.	Research	Conduct research that considers the influence of structures (not only behavior/ culture/ genetics) on health and healthcare

early career. Following the model of the previous arrow diagram, the structural factors influencing the provider's trajectory are then illustrated in red. Our hope was that this parallel arrow diagram – this time illustrating the structural influences on providers (including even relatively privileged providers) – would help make this section of the training "stickier" than it seemed to be in our pilot effort.

Based on our observations and evaluations of our subsequent iterations of the training, the above additions appeared to have the intended effects. Shirley's

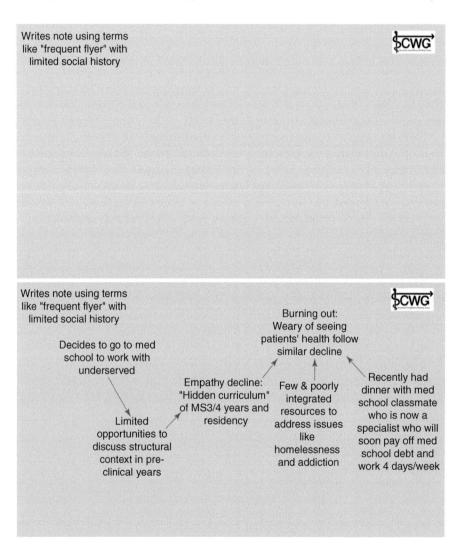

Fig. 3 Provider arrow diagram

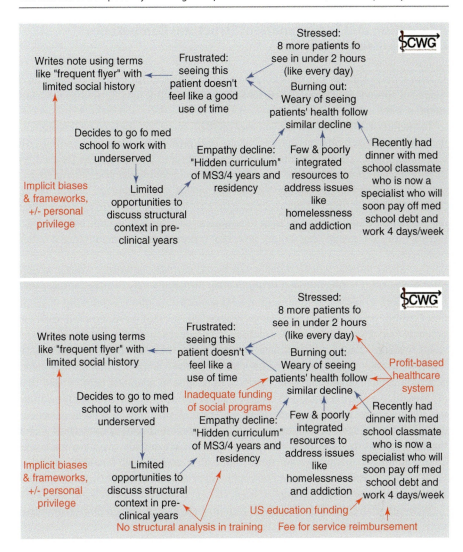

Fig. 3 (continued)

Beloved Community section and the examples of responses to structural issues were particularly popular. A number of participants commented that the "Levels of Intervention" helped them understand how they could implement structural competency into their work in the short term. And the addition of the provider arrow diagram appeared to make section two of the training "stickier" as hoped, as numerous participants commented on this diagram in post-training surveys.

Adaptation and Dissemination: Structural Competency for Diverse Audiences

In our second year, our group's experimentation and adaptation of the training for a variety of formats proliferated. See Table 1 above for a full list of training sites as of summer 2018.

In the fall of 2016 through the summer of 2017, the group focused on disseminating our training for others to utilize, adapt, and modify for their own settings. To accomplish this, we divided ourselves into subgroups. One subgroup focused on developing a training manual to provide context and training suggestions for educators and trainees who might view the training videos and introduce elements of the training to their institutions or other settings. Another subgroup explored in parallel the possibility of developing a "train the trainers" session, while a third developed a website for our group that could host the training videos, manual, and other resources.

This effort to disseminate the material raised various challenges. Aware of cultural competency's development in unintended directions – from its origins as a call for providers to recognize their cultural biases to its adoption as othering "lists of traits" to be memorized about various groups [20, 35, 36] – we wrestled with the potential for our materials and structural competency generally to be misunderstood, watered-down, and deployed in ways we would not support. With this in mind, we ultimately decided to abandon the "train the trainer" session development, concluding that we did not have capacity to do this in adequate depth – and that offering such a session could be perceived as our group endorsing the training abilities of those who participated. Instead, we are now planning to hold large, open-enrollment trainings once or twice yearly that interested parties can attend – and then bring what they desire to their own contexts. Meanwhile, we have made our 2016 training videos, trainer's manual, slide deck, and training handouts available to all on our website, www.structcomp.org. We are currently preparing our updated 2018 materials for dissemination.

With the wider distribution of our training, we expect our materials and message will be transformed – possibly for better as well as for worse. However, structural competency as a framework is rapidly gaining traction. Our hope is that the dissemination of materials such as these can contribute to structural competency maintaining a critical and meaningfully structural approach as it travels and grows.

Nuts and Bolts: Lessons About Group Structure

Before we close, in this section, we will share a few reflections about lessons we have learned over time about how to organize our group. For the first several years of its existence, the SCWG had minimal formal group structure. Initially, this informal approach worked well, as we were a small, committed group. We developed strong working relationships and came to know one another reasonably well. At any given time, one to three student members coordinated the group – planning and facilitating meetings, sending out emails, etc.

Gradually, however, the group's training became more widely known, and more people grew interested in joining us. At any given meeting, several new people would show up, many of whom would not sustain participation. It became ambiguous who was and was not in the group at any given time. As this happened, it became more challenging to conduct meetings and move projects forward. The informal approach that had worked for us initially seemed increasingly unsustainable.

To address these shortcomings, Shirley Strong and Josh Neff began developing a structure for the group, based on the organizational structure Josh had witnessed as a volunteer at the Berkeley Free Clinic. They created an application for new members, to complete after participating in at least one training. They requested a commitment of at least 1 year's involvement, with 6 hours total per month. They established a clear division of labor, with designated roles for various members (for instance, a website manager, a communications person, etc.). Finally, they created a process by which new members could become SCWG training facilitators. This process includes reading, writing about, and (at meetings) discussing a progression of articles and chapters and then helping lead portions of several trainings under the guidance of our group's established trainers.

Thus far, this new structure has restored a sense of momentum and accomplishment that the group had lost after its first few semesters. With this in place, the SCWG has recently been working in project-focused subgroups to better tailor the training to specific audiences, for instance, creating cases and other materials specific to reproductive health, mental health, and pre-health (undergraduate or high school) audiences. We have a highly motivated cohort of soon-to-be designated trainers who will be able to carry the group forward. Crucially, this new cohort represents a broad cross-section of professions and positionalities who are already bringing their various backgrounds and experiences to the training's ongoing development.

Conclusion: Core Lessons and Remaining Questions

At the start of this chapter, we framed several open questions about structural competency: to whom and how should structural competency be taught ("who" and "how") and which content should be highlighted ("what")? We will close by summarizing key insights into these questions that we gained from developing, implementing, evaluating, refining, and disseminating our structural competency training.

Who Our experience suggests that structural competency is potentially applicable to many disciplines. Providers across a variety of health fields – from nursing, medicine, and physical therapy to social work and even public health – responded favorably to our training, frequently expressing desire to incorporate structural competency into their practice. Furthermore, in a moment in which healthcare is striving to provide increasingly team-based and interprofessional care, it stands to reason that whole teams should be trained in structural competency. We have had positive experiences implementing trainings for both single-profession and interprofessional groups.

The reach of structural competency need not be limited to health practitioners; certainly cultural competency has been taken up well beyond its healthcare origins. We would propose that any field with professionally mediated contact with structurally vulnerable communities could benefit from structural competency training – for instance, teachers, attorneys, city planners, and environmental advocates, among many others.

Profession is just one axis to consider when contemplating the receptivity of various audiences to structural competency. Another variable is the political leanings of a given audience. The majority of our trainings have taken place in the relatively politically progressive Bay Area, so we are not able to speak to the ways that such content would be received in settings with different political climates.

It is notable, however, that our training was felt to be valuable in programs with reputations for being politically progressive. One might expect that structural competency training would be deemed redundant or unneeded in such settings, to the extent that progressive politics tend to highlight structural injustices. To the contrary, one month after participation in our training, SRFMR residents reported that they were "thinking about it constantly," that it was helping them "to build a partnership with patients," and that it made it "easier to talk about" structural issues with peers and faculty. Faculty comments post-training suggest that our training was of value even for long-time practitioners and clinical educators. As one faculty member put it, "I have a language and framework to use in something I have been teaching to residents for years without the language." We have received similarly positive responses at other sites at which we have conducted trainings.

We also have had experience running structural competency sessions with healthcare trainees at various stages of training. There have been minor modifications to our approach with participants at different stages – namely, creating more time for participants with significant clinical experience to share and process what they have encountered – but for the most part, we have delivered the same training. Based on our experience facilitating these sessions, the reactions have been more or less similar across stages of training, with the exception that pre-clinical trainees tend to request more explanation of how the content at hand is relevant to their field when compared to participants with greater clinical experience.

How We found that thinking about what would be "sticky" for clinicians was helpful in developing and refining the pedagogy of our training. By pushing ourselves to think in these terms, we designed sessions distinct from the usual presentation of social science content. While it is challenging to present such material in a fashion that most will find engaging, it is even more challenging to present in a way that the content will be remembered by participants more than a day or a week afterward. To achieve this, we employed visuals (including our "arrow diagrams"), case-based pedagogy, and a minimum of technical social-scientific jargon, as well as providing repeated opportunities for reflection and interaction. This combination of techniques appears to have been effective, as a month afterward participants reported thinking about the content we introduced "constantly." In addition, the brevity of these trainings – generally three hours – pushed us to be clear and focus on the most essential, potentially "sticky" points that we wanted to impart to participants.

We continue to strive to balance the didactic sections of our training with the interactive and reflective elements. We are often asked to condense the training into one or two hour sessions to fit into available time slots, which restricts the time available for interaction and reflection. Post-training, we often get feedback that participants would like more time for the training, and particularly for the interactive portions. We continue to believe, however, that the didactic portions of the training are indispensable, given limited time and that we are attempting to promote a common vocabulary among participants.

As far as the "how" of our group organization, we have had to adjust our approach as our work and our group have developed. While we initially had success with an informal group process, over time we have found it beneficial to develop a clear group structure. Among the most important aspects of this structure were requesting a specific commitment from new group members, establishing a clearer division of labor, and developing a process by which new group members could become SCWG "trainers." We think and hope that this structure will help the group to be sustainable and maintain diversity over time.

What In our experience, *structural violence* has been a powerful and "sticky" concept. Perhaps this is inherently so for healthcare professionals, to the extent this lens helps us as providers to better understand the health and experiences of patients with whom we work on a day-to-day basis. Though initially less "sticky" than structural violence, with revisions, *naturalizing inequality* has also become a concept that trainees report influencing their thinking. Several participants noted that they found our discussion of the relationships among structural competency, cultural competency, and the social determinants of health crucial as well, noting that these distinctions clarified what it means to develop a structural analysis of health and healthcare.

Time and again in the evaluations, participants' expressed a strong desire to intervene to change harmful social structures. In some cases, this desire to intervene has been paired with distress about uncertainty as to how to do so. To address this, we have included more historical and contemporary examples of how clinicians and others have responded to structural issues; subsequent participants have expressed appreciation for this portion. We also began emphasizing the various possible "levels of intervention," which participants have reported has helped them feel able to begin taking action based on a structural perspective.

These modifications are not adequate to resolve all participants' distress at social and health inequities. In fact, as noted earlier, we feel that some distress is an appropriate response when confronting the extent of the suffering that results from unjust social structures. Furthermore, we suspect that a degree of distress may motivate health professionals to partake in efforts to address harmful structures. However, we know how overwhelming healthcare training and practice can be, and we do not wish to contribute to this burden. To help prevent participants from feeling overwhelmed, we now close our trainings by discussing and attempting to normalize a range of possible reactions, from distress and overwhelm to inspiration and motivation. We also attempt to speak to the fact that – while many healthcare practitioners, whether due to training or disposition, wish to take individual action and see discrete outcomes – structural issues require collective responses. Such collective action often involves following the leadership of others, and change develops over unpredictable timeframes. Ideally, we hope to promote a sense of working to address structural issues over "the long haul" – which means making peace with being structurally humble and not necessarily getting immediate results, as well as trying to avoid overextending oneself and thereby increasing the likelihood of burning out.

In the United States and around the world, social, political, and economic structures are hugely determinant of the distribution of illness and health. Structural competency is a promising framework to help clinicians recognize, analyze, ameliorate, and hopefully alter these harmful inequities. To bring this framework to health professionals, the Structural Competency Working Group has developed, operationalized, evaluated, and revised a three hour structural competency training. Encouraging "impractical" innovative thinking, striving to make content "sticky," and responding to findings from evaluation, the SCWG developed a brief training that we have found to be surprisingly impactful. Our efforts to implement and evaluate this training for a variety of healthcare professions suggest that it can be similarly relevant across a range of fields.

We hope our case will inspire others to implement similar trainings in other geographical locations and for professionals in other fields – within and beyond healthcare. One of the benefits of structural competency training that emerged in our evaluations was the development of shared language and frameworks among colleagues. We think that structural competency has potential to foster a similar phenomenon at a larger scale, promoting a shared structural language and orientation within entire disciplines and, ultimately, across various sectors of society. And we believe that providing this foundation is a key step toward developing a movement in which we can work together to realize a more equal, healthy, and just future.

Acknowledgments The Structural Competency Working Group's efforts have been supported by the Berkeley Center for Social Medicine and Deborah Lustig as well as the University of California Humanities Research Institute.

Josh Neff's work on this project has been supported by the UCSF Resource Allocation Program for Trainees (RAPtr), the Greater Good Science Center Hornaday Fellowship, UC Berkeley-UCSF Joint Medical Program Thesis Grant, and the Helen Marguerite Schoeneman Scholarship.

References

1. Morris LT, Roush C, Spencer LE. The arc of the universe is long: Unitarian Universalists, anti-racism, and the journey from Calgary. Skinner House Books. 2009. 651 p.
2. Geiger J. Community health centers: health care as an instrument of social change. In: Sidel VW, Sidel R, editors. Reforming medicine: lessons of the last quarter century. New York: Pantheon Books; 1984.
3. Holmes SM, Ponte M. En-case-ing the patient : disciplining uncertainty in medical student patient presentations. Cult Med Psychiatry. 2011;35(2):163–82.
4. Metzl JM, Hansen H. Structural competency: theorizing a new medical engagement with stigma and inequality. Soc Sci Med. Elsevier Ltd. 2014;103:126–33.
5. Pine A. From healing to witchcraft: on ritual speech and roboticization in the hospital. Cult Med Psychiatry. 2011;35:262–84.
6. Rivkin-Fish M. Learning the moral economy of commodified health care: "community education," failed consumers, and the shaping of ethical clinician-citizens. Cult Med Psychiatry. 2011;35(2):183–208.
7. Nazar M, Kendall K, Day L, Nazar H. Decolonising medical curricula through diversity education: lessons from students. Med Teach. Informa Healthcare. 2015;37(4):385–93.
8. Kumagai AK, Lypson ML. Beyond cultural competence: critical consciousness, social justice, and multicultural education. Acad Med. 2009;84(6):782–7.
9. Paul D, Ewen SC, Jones R. Cultural competence in medical education: aligning the formal, informal and hidden curricula. Adv Heal Sci Educ. Springer Netherlands. 2014;19(5):751–8.
10. Smith WR, Betancourt JR, Wynia MK, Bussey-Jones J, Stone VE, Phillips CO, et al. Recommendations for teaching about racial and ethnic disparities in health and health care. Ann Intern Med. American College of Physicians. 2007;147(9):654.
11. Quesada J, Arreola S, Kral A, Khoury S, Organista KC, Worby P. "As good as it gets": undocumented Latino day laborers negotiating discrimination in San Francisco and Berkeley, California, USA. City Soc (Wash). NIH Public Access. 2014;26(1):29–50.
12. Farmer PE, Nizeye B, Stulac S, Keshavjee S. Structural violence and clinical medicine. PLoS Med [Internet]. 2006;3(10):e449.
13. Bourgois P. Recognizing invisible violence: a thirty-year ethnographic retrospective. In: Rylko-Bauer B, Whiteford L, Farmer P, editors. Global health in times of violence. Santa Fe: School for Advanced Research Press; 2009. p. 17–40.
14. Quesada J, Hart LK, Bourgois P. Structural vulnerability and health: Latino migrant laborers in the United States. Med Anthropol. 2012;30(4):1–17.
15. Bourgois P, Holmes SM, Sue K, Quesada J. Structural vulnerability. Acad Med [Internet]. 2016 Jul 12.
16. Holmes SM. An ethnographic Study of the Social Context of Migrant Health in the United States. Gill P, editor. PLoS Med. Public Library of Science. 2006;3(10):e448.
17. Wacquant L. Pierre Bourdieu. In: Key sociological thinkers. London: Macmillan; 1998. p. 215–29.
18. Burawoy M. The roots of domination: beyond bourdieu and gramsci. Sociology. 2012;46:187–206.
19. Gregg J, Saha S. Losing culture on the way to competence : the use and misuse of culture in medical. Acad Med. 2006;81(6):542–7.
20. Jenks AC. From "lists of traits" to "open-mindedness": emerging issues in cultural competence education. Cult Med Psychiatry [Internet]. 2011;35(2):209–35.
21. Marmot M. Social determinants of health inequalities. Lancet [Internet]. 2005 Jan [cited 2014 Sep 11];365(9464):1099–104.
22. Marmot M. The health gap: doctors and the social determinants of health. Scand J Public Health [Internet]. SAGE Publications Sage UK: London, England; 2017 Nov 22.
23. Krieger N. A glossary for social epidemiology. J Epidemiol Community Health [Internet]. BMJ Publishing Group Ltd; 2001 Oct 1.

24. Krieger N. Proximal, distal, and the politics of causation: what's level got to do with it?. Am J Public Health [Internet]. American Public Health Association; 2008 Feb 10.
25. Harvey M, McGladrey M. Explaining the origins and distribution of health and disease: an analysis of epidemiologic theory in core Master of Public Health coursework in the United States. Crit Public Health. 2018:1–13.
26. McKenna B, Baer H. Dying for capitalism. Counterpunch. August 02, 2012.
27. Boler M. Chapter 7: teaching for hope the ethics of shattering world views. In: Liston DP, Garrison JW, editors. Teaching, learning, and loving: reclaiming passion in educational practice. New York: RoutledgeFalmer; 2004.
28. Wear D, Aultman JM. The limits of narrative: Medical student resistance to confronting inequality and oppression in literature and beyond. Medical Educ. 2005;39:1056–65.
29. Willen SS. Confronting a "Big Huge Gaping Wound": emotion and anxiety in a cultural sensitivity course for psychiatry residents. Cult Med Psychiatry. 2013;37(2):253–79.
30. Aiken LH, Cimiotti JP, Sloane DM, Smith HL, Flynn L, Neff DF. Effects of nurse staffing and nurse education on patient deaths in hospitals with different nurse work environments. Med Care. NIH Public Access. 2011;49(12):1047–53.
31. Aiken LH, Sloane DM, Bruyneel L, Van den Heede K, Griffiths P, Busse R, et al. Nurse staffing and education and hospital mortality in nine European countries: a retrospective observational study. Lancet. Elsevier. 2014; 383(9931):1824–1830.
32. Neff J, Knight KR, Satterwhite S, Nelson N, Matthews J, Holmes SM. Teaching structure: a qualitative evaluation of a structural competency training for resident physicians. J Gen Intern Med. 2017;32(4):430–3.
33. Nelson A. Longue Durée of black lives matter, Am J Public Health. American Public Health Association. 2016;106(10):1734–7.
34. Messac L, Ciccarone D, Draine J, Bourgois P. The good-enough science-and-politics of anthropological collaboration with evidence-based clinical research: Four ethnographic case studies. Soc Sci Med. Elsevier Ltd. 2013;99:176–86.
35. Tervalon M, Murray-Garcia J. Cultural humility versus cultural competence. J Health Care Poor Underserved. 1998;9(2):117–25.
36. Kleinman A, Benson P. Anthropology in the clinic: the problem of cultural competency and how to fix it. PLoS Med. 2006;3(10):e294.

Teaching Social Medicine as Collaborative Ethnographic Research and Advocacy on Homelessness and Serious Mental Illness

Joel T. Braslow and Philippe Bourgois

The Problem: How Can Social Science Methods and Theory Engage Theoretically and Practically in the US Medical School Context with the Urgent Challenges of Rising Social Inequality and Health Disparities

Health, disease, health-care delivery, and medical science are deeply shaped by social, political, economic, and cultural structures [1]. Critical social science perspectives, however, remain underdeveloped in US medical schools. A growing number medical schools are promoting versions of "social medicine" and devoting more curricular time to "cultural competence", "social determinants of health" [2], and "structural competence" [3–5], but most of this curriculum is taught by clinicians without graduate-level social science training and does not systematically integrate the methods and theories of medical social sciences. As two of only a handful of senior social scientists on the faculty of the medical school at the UCLA, we have taken it upon ourselves (with encouragement from a progressive dean's office) to develop ways of incorporating social science methods and theory into both the undergraduate medical school curriculum as well as the larger intellectual community of clinical researchers, postdocs, fellows, and clinicians throughout the medical school. This also involves increasing interdisciplinary linkages between the medical school and social science and humanities departments across campus.

J. T. Braslow (✉)
UCLA David Geffen School of Medicine, University of California, Los Angeles, Los Angeles, CA, USA
e-mail: Jbraslow@ucla.edu

P. Bourgois (✉)
Semel Institute of Neuroscience, Department Psychiatry and Biobehavioral Sciences, David Geffen School of Medicine, University of California, Los Angeles, Los Angeles, CA, USA
e-mail: bourgois@ucla.edu

© Springer Nature Switzerland AG 2019
H. Hansen, J. M. Metzl (eds.), *Structural Competency in Mental Health and Medicine*,
https://doi.org/10.1007/978-3-030-10525-9_6

Our guiding questions are: (1) how can we build social medicine as a discipline and vibrant intellectual community in a public medical school that goes beyond its standard, well-intentioned but only token presence within the curriculum; and (2) how can we integrate critical thinking about the impacts of social forces on health into the very fabric of medical education, intellectual socialization, clinical practice, research, and advocacy? We believe that social medicine ought to encompass a larger epistemological and moral frame, one that allows for a critical self-reflexive engagement with both medicine and society and become the basis for a vision of research and clinical practice dedicated to social justice for structurally vulnerable populations. As a medical anthropologist (PB) and a medical historian and psychiatrist (JB), we share a sensibility for the importance of understanding the historical, social, and cultural context of our objects of study as well as our own prejudices. We both also want to make sense of Los Angeles, the community we live in, through a theoretical and practical understanding of how social structural forces shape social inequality and damage the health and life chances of vulnerable underserved populations. Arguably the sprawling suburbanized megalopolis of Los Angeles is the global city of the future, incubating many of the most dramatic structural inequities facing the United States.In fact, social contradictions and suffering becomes exceptionally visible in our city because of its large and exaggerated scale. In fact historically, political, economic, and sociocultural trends in California, primarily driven by Los Angeles, the most populous county in the nation have presaged future developments across the country. In recent generations this has ranged from the 1960s countercultural hippie peace/love/sexual liberation movements and legistlation of civil liberty protections, to the 1978 right-wing populist taxpayer revolt of proposition 13 that contributed to the 1980 presidential election of Ronald Reagan and set the US on the path to punitive neoliberalism [6] followed by a series of legislative "reforms" that resulted in the state of California having the fastest rising rates of mass incarceration during peacetime of any nation in world history from 1980 through the mid-1990s [7].

We both live on the Westside of the city near campus, where average house values exceed $1.5 million. This inflated opulence, however, is undone by – and comes at the cost of – nearly 50,000 homeless individuals in Los Angeles County, many of whom call the streets, alleys, and freeway underpasses surrounding us their home.

We either walk (JB) or bicycle (PB) to work and are bombarded daily with the contradictions of dramatic social inequality besetting our city. We each pass dozens of homeless individuals on our separate short commutes to and from work. We catch ourselves reflexively avoiding eye contact when we pass distressed individuals who often find themselves in frantic states of florid psychotic decompensation or paralyzed by despair. Despite our personal political, intellectual, and professional proclivities, and despite our multiple publications on the structural policy and economic forces promoting homelessness at the daily level, we de facto reproduce society's growing indifference to the rising levels of social suffering and survival insecurity that is imposed on increasing numbers of our homeless, often seriously mentally ill, neighbors [6, 8, 9]. Survey data estimates that only some 30% of the Los Angeles homeless population suffers from serious mental illness [10] but they are the most visible of all the homeless, marked by the accumulated dirt and grime embedded in their rags and skin and by their frequently odd public behaviors. One does not need psychiatric training to know that their mental illness is inseparable from their homelessness. Ironically our offices are located on the ground floor of UCLA's repurposed neuropsychiatric hospital that was opened in 1961 as a subsidized therapeutic facility during the golden age of public mental health that would have considered our current practice of abandoning to the streets or incarcerating those afflicted with psychosis to be a barbaric relic of early nineteenth century practices. The old state-funded neuropsychiatric hospital, however, has succumbed to the invisible hand of neoliberalism. Rechristened the Stewart and Lynda Resnick Neuropsychiatric Hospital after billionaire philanthropists who offset dwindling state support with a sizable gift, the hospital no longer regularly cares for the indigent. It has changed its priorities to serving patients with private health insurance. Relocated within the newly built and aptly neoliberally named Ronald Reagan Medical Center, the ostensibly public the Resnick Neuropsychiatric Hospital boasts a US News and World Report ranking of 8th in psychiatric hospitals, but it is off-limits to the sickest, most vulnerable homeless indigent individuals with serious mental illness. They can be seen every day, wandering the streets and alleyways surrounding the hospital, often in states of unimaginable terror and distress. All too often they are forcibly removed or shoo-ed away by police or security guards. Nevertheless, along with our clinical colleagues we routinely ignore and avoid them.

Theoretical Orientation

More of a perspective than a grand theoretical orientation, we both seek to understand the ways in which larger political economic forces underpin relationships of power and how those relationships, in turn, shape social, cultural, and psychological life. This critical social science approach, combined with our everyday context of living in Los Angeles has shaped our appraoch to training medical students and residents. We see the city as a natural laboratory for critiquing the negative health effects of rising levels of social inequality, financialization of public resources and policy planning and implementation that promotes segregated gentrification processes.

Year after year, we have been amazed at the idealism, enthusiasm, and fundamental humanism animating many, if not most, of the entering classes of medical students. As these same students progress through their medical training, however, they steadily lose (or misplace) their commitments to social justice. We believe that social medicine teaching, no matter how one conceives of it, should foster and protect this early idealism and provide a productive analytical framework that helps students mature into socially responsible physicians and/or researchers committed to a broader notion of health, social equality, and solidarity for the suffering imposed on structurally vulnerable populations by social forces and policies.

Our views on medical education fit into how we hope to more generally situate our scholarship. We aspire to being public intellectuals or, more humbly, "good-enough [11] specific intellectuals [11]" to meld the provocatively self-critical terms of Nancy Scheper-Hughes [11] and Foucault [12, 13]. We share a political and intellectual commitment to bringing the methods and theory of a critical social science of medicine approach to bear on the urgent social problems of the larger community surrounding us and what we see as the central or emerging contradictions of our historical era plagued by rising local and global social inequality. We hope that both us and our students become more than bystanders in the face of contemporary inequalities and rise to the challenge of helping to create a medical practice and research that reflects these values that originally inspired JB to become a physician and PB to develop social medicine training programs in medical schools.

The Path

Reproducing Ourselves

Since the late 1990s, each of us has been building social medicine programs in medical schools (at the University of California, San Francisco; the University of California, Berkeley; the University of Pennsylvania; and now together at the University of California, Los Angeles). In each setting, we have had distinct institutional homes – as a full department with dedicated hard-money faculty salaries at the University of California as San Francisco and Berkeley, as a doctoral program track with only part-time faculty within a larger social science department and a fledgling public health program at the University of Pennsylvania, and as a center with both full-time and part-time faculty at UCLA who are appointed in multiple departments across campus and public sector agencies in the city (Department of Mental Health) and the region (Veterans Associations). The overarching goals of our programs, however, have changed little over the years: namely, to build an intellectual community of researchers, students, and clinicians dedicated to bringing the methods and theories of a critical social science of medicine approach to bear on understanding how social inequality impacts health, caregiving, and scientific knowledge.

Despite the very distinct institutional settings and funding streams of each of our social medicine programs over the years, they have been anchored by MD/PhD training programs funded with support from NIH Medical Scientist Training Program (MSTP), supplemented by sometimes generous dean's offices as well as an unstable scramble of public and private grants and elusive philanthropy. This has enabled us to admit 1–3 doctoral students per year to an interdisciplinary cross-school 9-year program that supports integrated MD (4 years) and PhD (4.5–5 years) training in the social sciences/humanities (primarily anthropology, sociology, and history in our cases). The exceptional intelligence, discipline, and appeal of these students and – more practically – their guaranteed funding and tendency towards ambitious over-achievement facilitates our engagement with the larger intellectual community of social science PhD programs across the campus. Most practically it attracts new interdisciplinary faculty colleagues eager to serve as mentors and members of a social medicine intellectual community who often become excellent unpaid faculty affiliates in our Center. The MD/PhD students rise to the challenge of merging theoretical perspectives and practices from the medical and social sciences. This seemingly intractable epistemological contradiction spawns what can be called (following Bourdieu, 2008 [14]) a productive "fractured [disciplinary/vocational clinician-social scientist] habitus" that makes these budding MD/PhDs reflexively uncomfortable (on both conscious analytical and also preconscious emotional levels) in the two occupational worlds (clinical practice versus social science academia) that organize their lives, shape their intellectual maturation processes, and fund them. Their simultaneous training in multiple contradictory epistemological worlds sometimes promotes exceptionally creative – what Bourdieu would call "non-doxic" – critical thinking [15]. Most of the trainees pursue careers in academic medicine informed by their critical social science perspective but also committed to practical professional engagement with caregiving. This often pushes those that do not become seduced or distracted by the exceptionally high salaries paid to US practitioners to challenge the accepted status quo boundaries of thinking among their colleagues within their distinct institutional settings. At all four universities where we have worked, the social medicine program did not flower until it benefited from the MD/PhD training program which provided funding, symbolic institutional legitimization, and a logistics of practical collaboration fomenting faculty collegiality.

Our MD/PhD students repeatedly prod us to engage formally with the existing undergraduate medical school curriculum. This is especially the case during their first 2 years of medical school, when they are excited about trying on their new dual identities of social scientist and physician. Medical education claims to be moving away from rote memorization, but standardized national certification exams structure the learning and teaching experience and our social science and social justice-oriented students find little in their formal medical curriculum to address their interest in the social context of disease or health disparities. As a result, the MD/PhD students often spontaneously develop social medicine pedagogical initiatives on their own. They often become lecturers, trainers of small group preceptors, and even organizers of entire courses or thematic threads within the undergraduate medical school curriculum [16]. Again, their unique positionality as medical-student-socialscientists-in-training at the frontlines of social medicine pedagogy offers us insiders' participant-observation perspectives on the "pulse" of changing generational sensibilities of medical students towards critical thinking. Our students, independently from us, enrich the intellectual environment of the medical school and motivate other students to pursue their commitments to health and social equality. Some have even gone on to found or lead political advocacy and physician/social scientist disciplinary organizations [17].

Social Medicine for All

Despite the pedagogical enthusiasm of many of our MD/PhD students, developing and administering a core required curriculum in social medicine for all MD students remains an unachieved challenge for us. Medical student teaching is poorly rewarded institutionally. Furthermore, staking out territory for social medicine in an already crowded clinical curriculum often riddled with alpha personalities convinced, like us of the universal importance of their particular medical/intellectual sub-disciplines is a thankless task.

Medical schools are notorious for repeatedly "reinventing" their curriculum but failing to achieve substantial change. Indeed our experience with introducing social medicine into those ambitious curriculum-wide overhauls have often felt like excercises in slamming our heads against brick walls. Over our years of fits and starts, we have organized multiple social science initiatives to energize our emerging intellectual community of social medicine practitioners and researchers and to increase its size, diversity, relevance, and presence in pedagogy throughout our medical school. These initiatives have in the past included or are in the process of hopefully becoming: (1) a social medicine thread of strategic lectures and small group sessions in the required first-year doctoring course; (2) a 2-week social medicine block in the first year of medical school followed by a longitudinal component that threads through all 4 years; (3) short elective courses for medical students offered in the first-year, fourth-year, and over summer sessions; (4) taskforces of faculty members from across campus to propose and revise – yet again! – the core social medicine curriculum and redefine cultural competency as "cultural humility" and/or [18] structural competency [4]; (5) bimonthly social medicine seminars organized around social science readings relevant to our current research projects that attract medical students, MD/PhD and social science graduate students, postdocs, residents, and faculty; (6) a quarterly social medicine grand round series; (7) social science clinical case conference series; (8) positions as attending social scientists in clinical case conference series within hospital residency training programs in which the residents present patients whose conditions are complicated by social conditions in which we have some expertise (such as psychosis, substance use disorder, homelessness, incarceration); (9) monthly clinical self-reflexive ethnographic fieldnote methods seminars; and (10) introducing "structural vulnerability" checklists [5] to residencies to adapt and implement within their specific clinical settings, community social services resource bases and larger social structural risk environments.

Engaging the Social

Over the last few years, somewhat more humbly and/or opportunistically, we have aligned our teaching more closely with our research commitments and policy engagement. This has the immediate practical advantage of reducing the double-bind of the zero-sum time conflict between teaching, research and unstable research funding and engages us spontaneously into conveying inadvertently our passion for a social medicine that addresses urgent health disparities and social problems. Our current research commitments, for example, arise directly out of our daily passage through the contradictory landscape of growing social inequality, homelessness, and indigent serious mental illness in our rapidly gentrifying city. Just as tragically and structurally inseparable from its levels of homelessness, Los Angeles law enforcement agencies arrest and incarcerate more seriously mentally ill individuals than any other city on the planet. The Los Angeles County Jail has become the largest de facto psychiatric institution in the world according to the United Nations [19], with between 4000 and 5000 seriously mentally ill inmates behind bars on any given day, with many of them floridly decompensating in solitary cells. Starting first as a trickle in the 1970s and then, over the last 40 years, becoming a torrent, people with serious mental illness have been increasingly churned into intractable cycles of homelessness, acute hospitalization, and incarceration. From 2009 through 2018 the absolute and relative number of Los Angeles County Jail inmates with serious mental illness increased 80 percent [20–22]. We have worked together to understand the larger structural political economic forces and the specific changing regional policy initiatives that inadvertently sustain this nefarious cycle of institutionalized suffering in our sprawling megalopolis. We are documenting how these macro-level forces and the systems-level fragmentation of public and private safety net agencies translate into the intimate experience of everyday suffering, despair and serious mental and physical illness?

Although we had often collaborated closely with individual MD/PhDs and other social science graduate students on specific research projects in the past, we initially conceived of our current collaborative team research as being largely separate from – and in zero-sum time competition with — our pedagogical interests in and obligations to undergraduate medical school education. Generally, our multiple formal teaching initiatives have tended to burn us out, sabotaging their effectiveness in practically modeling to our students the practicality of sustainable socially responsible practices on behalf of underserved populations in academic medicine. Partially out of frustration, consequently, we experimented with aligning our teaching more closely with our personal research commitments. JB had just obtained a large contract to evaluate a program administered by the Los Angeles County Department of Mental Health (LACDMH) to address the growing problem of individuals cycling through homelessness, acute psychiatric hospitalization, arrest and incarceration. We were excitedly scrambling to find time and personnel to develop a multi-method, clinically informed quantitative/qualitative/ethnographic evaluation that would explicitly link larger social forces to everyday suffering and disease: the essence of our (perhaps idiosyncratic) critical definition of social medicine around political economic power vectors.

Theory and Practice: Teaching Social Medicine as Applied Sociomedical Practice

We began by killing two birds with one stone and subordinated a required first-year medical student teaching module under the priorities our new applied research effort. We developed a 6-week summer elective that took advantage of existing medical school stipends available to first-year medical students transitioning into second year who were seeking to temporarily apprentice on existing faculty research projects. We also integrated two incoming members of our class of social science track MD/PhDs who already had formal undergraduate training in the social sciences and were familiar with ethnographic qualitative methods. They served as peer leaders for the less experienced medical students. We organized the theme of the elective as an exploratory "ethnographic diagnostic overview" of the unmet mental and physical health needs of the homeless in Los Angeles.

We began with a very brief theoretical training in the historical, social, and political economic context of inequality and homelessness in Los Angeles. The bulk of those introductory sessions focused practically on the logistics of participant-observation ethnographic methods and the sensibilities of critical self-reflection and cultural relativism. Most importantly, at the end of the first class, both faculty members accompanied the students to conduct an evening of fieldwork in a homeless encampment two blocks from our classroom where JB had developed some friendly acquaintances. The faculty members wrote up the first draft of that evening's ethnographic field note. The students then added their additional observations on subsequent drafts, with each student using a different colored text to identify their positionality and voice. This collaborative technique became the model for the collaborative group ethnography over the next 6 weeks. They went on fieldwork outings in pairs with one of the students taking the lead in writing the field note and the other adding observations to the original note. Sometimes one of us or a faculty member or the ethnographer staff member (Ronald Calderon) from our Center accompanied them, providing a third experienced perspective, as well as facilitating ongoing logistical coordination and local institutional or community-entre to new sites. The notes were posted to a HIPAA compliant server, and we all met once a week to discuss our findings, emerging hypotheses, and brainstorm future sites for fieldwork and for supplemental archival data collection.

The Key Learning

This tentative experiment exceeded our expectations. The medical students enthusiastically fanned out across the city to strategically selected distinct urban ecologies of Los Angeles where large populations of homeless congregate: Skid Row, West Hollywood, sex strolls, Venice, the Boardwalk, MacArthur Park in East Los Angeles, and Veterans Park in Westwood. Smart, motivated medical students make excellent ethnographers. Their non-threatening positionality as eager-to-learn youth, not yet jaded by long hours of clinical call or dispiriting hierarchies of hospital life, facilitate sympathetic access to a diverse range of often overwhelmed social service providers, stakeholders and homeless individuals who are sometimes distrustful of academic clinical researchers. Even conservative police officers openly hostile to the politics of public health and social science researchers let down their guard and opened up generously to the students inviting them to shadow them on patrols.

At the same time, the quality of their clinically informed and anthropology-inspired, culturally relative field notes caught us by surprise. They became a useful set of comparative field notes that triangulated multiple political perspectives and ethnic/class/gender/sexuality positionalities. Their field notes on difficult-to-engage street settings including gang-controlled drug-selling scenes became a valuable part of our applied research/service data archive.

The students also bonded intellectually as a cohort through the intensity of the experience of street-based fieldwork among indigent vulnerable populations on unfamiliar social turf. In fact, in subsequent years, these students became a new set of core participants of our applied social medicine intellectual community, eager to bring their skills to bear on the urgent social problems in our surrounding community or in the larger global environment. The students told us that the ethnographic practicum was the first time they had engaged in a substantial manner with the larger Los Angeles community from which they had felt isolated during their first year. They were moved by the stakes of the suffering they encountered on the street. This gave them a sense of the possibility of becoming clinicians on behalf of the underserved. It opened their imagination to longer-term career commitments in social medicine, public service, and health and social service including political and clinical advocacy. They urged us to scale up this kind of participant observation in an applied, community-based, and clinical/social science research/service opportunity and even argued that all the medical students in their class should be required to engage in projects led by multiple different research coordinators in local or global contexts.

On a more personal level, each of the summer ethnographers admitted to having experienced a creeping, corrosive alienation during their first year of classroom learning that distanced them from the values of medicine as a healing vocation that had attracted them to medical school in the first place. A couple of the students even confessed to having considered dropping out of medical school during their first year of coursework because of the disconnect between what they were being taught in the classroom and their commitments to social justice as well as their everyday experience of inequality in Los Angeles. They all expressed relief at having finally found a community of open-minded progressive "fellow travelers" in the otherwise competitive sprint through medical school. Indeed, through their next year of coursework, they continued to meet with one another and attend many of our bimonthly social medicine seminars and quarterly grand rounds. We furnished a set of cubicle alcoves for medical students and they began hanging out in our Center for Social Medicine office space alongside the MD/PhDs. They even started a basketball team and practiced on the court outside of our center's offices. Several of them went on to take leadership in student organizations and in free clinics for the homeless affiliated with UCLA again completely independent from us.

Emerging Projects and Lessons Learned

While we have not completely given up on creating a core, didactic required curriculum of social medicine for all medical students, we realize that it is a limited goal that may not be as impactful as we might like it to be. Despite a few notable exceptions, stable social medicine programs in medical schools [23] remain anomalies dependent upon soft money and the personal charisma of leadership. Social medicine will never be as central a part of medical school life, values, and epistemology as are the basic laboratory and clinical sciences. Our practical ethnographic experiment with the summer group medical student practicum of clinically informed ethnography demonstrated to us that social medicine needs to be seen as both a theory and a clinical practice, where everyday suffering must be accessed experientially with humility for it to be documented, explored theoretically and hopefully ultimately engaged with practically and sustainably.

We have continued to initiate team ethnographies on applied research projects with medical students and expanded it to include clinical residents and additional clinical faculty. Most recently, this includes documenting the wounds, scars and life stories of Central American refugees in the migrant caravan who are seeking asylum from organized crime but have become trapped in temporary detainment camps in Tijuana. We also continue our more labor-intensive pedagogical efforts with new cohorts of medical students expanding it to include clinical residents. Most productive has been our extension of ethnographic experiential training in nonclinical settings to residents. In the Department of Psychiatry, for example, residents have worked with us to initiate a formal clinical rotation in the Los Angeles County Jail's Mental Health Unit. This is a collaboration with the Department of Health Services' Correctional Health Services Unit that delivers all health services in the nation's largest County jail. This psychiatric rotation will also include a once a month afternoon session of clinical field note circulation and discussion to reflect on the contradictions and limits to therapeutic care in a carceral setting. This rotation cum ethnographic reflection protocol originated from field trips we have been taking with psychiatry residents in the county jail and their disorientation at the shock of witnessing face-to-face the routinized institutional violence of the criminalization of psychotic illness in contemporary California.

As we continue to explore how we might bring our pedagogical research practicums to scale, we continue to learn from and be inspired by the energy of our students and clinical trainees. They have reinvigorated our pleasure in teaching and mentoring by breaking the zero-sum contradiction between research and teaching. Though obvious to us in retrospect, we have learned that the most effective way to teach social medicine more sustainably in a way that reinforces idealistic commitments to social justice is to engage students in the same social and medical research problems and urgent human existential contradictions that animate our research.

References

1. Stonington S, Holmes SM. Social medicine in the twenty-first century. PLoS Med [Internet]. 2006 Oct;3(10). Available from: https://www.ncbi.nlm.nih.gov/pmc/articles/PMC1621097/
2. Marmot M, Allen J, Bell R, Bloomer E, Goldblatt P, Consortium for the European Review of Social Determinants of Health and the Health Divide. WHO European review of social determinants of health and the health divide. Lancet. 2012;380(9846):1011–29.
3. Association of American Medical Colleges [Internet]. Washington, DC: Association of American Medical Colleges; 2005. Cultural Competence Education for Medical Students. Available from: https://www.aamc.org/download/54338/data/
4. Hansen H, Braslow J, Rohrbaugh RM. From cultural to structural competency-training psychiatry residents to act on social determinants of health and institutional racism. JAMA Psychiat. 2018;75(2):117–8.
5. Bourgois P, Holmes SM, Sue K, Quesada J. Structural vulnerability: operationalizing the concept to address health disparities in clinical care. Acad Med. 2017;92(3):299–307.
6. Bourgois P, Schonberg J. Righteous dopefiend. 1st ed. Berkeley: University of California Press; 2009.

7. Zimring FE, Hawkins G. The growth of imprisonment in California. Br J Criminol. 1994;34(S1):83–96. https://doi.org/10.1093/oxfordjournals.bjc.34.S1.83.

8. Braslow J, Marder SR. History of Psychopharmacology. Annual Review of Clinical Psychology. 2019. https://www.annualreviews.org/clinpsy/planned

9. Braslow J. Mental ills and bodily cures: psychiatric treatment in the first half of the twentieth century. 1st ed. Berkeley: University of California Press; 1997.

10. Los Angeles Homeless Services Authority. Los Angeles Homeless Services Authority Homeless Count 2019 Report. [Internet]. Los Angeles; 2019. https://www.lahsa.org/homeless-count/

11. Scheper-Hughes N. Death without weeping: the violence of everyday life in Brazil. 1st ed. Berkeley: University of California Press; 1993.

12. Foucault M. In: Gordon C, editor. Power/knowledge: selected interviews and other writings, 1972–1977. 1st American ed. New York: Vintage; 1980.

13. Messac L, Ciccarone D, Draine J, Bourgois P. The good-enough science-and-politics of anthropological collaboration with evidence-based clinical research: four ethnographic case studies. Soc Sci Med. 2013;99:176–86.

14. Bourdieu P. Homo academicus. 1st ed. Stanford: Stanford University Press; 1990.

15. Bourdieu P. Outline of a theory of practice. 1st English ed. Cambridge: Cambridge University Press; 1977.

16. Dao DK, Goss AL, Hoekzema AS, et al. Integrating theory, content, and method to foster critical consciousness in medical students: a comprehensive model for cultural competence training. Acad Med. 2017;92(3):335–44.

17. Holmes SM, Karlin J, Stonington SD, Gottheil DL. The first nationwide survey of MD-PhDs in the social sciences and humanities: training patterns and career choices. BMC Med Educ. 2017;17(1):60.

18. Tervalon M, Murray-García J. Cultural humility versus cultural competence. J Health Care Poor Underserved. 1998;9(2):117–25.

19. World Health Organization [WHO]. Beds in general hospitals for mental health and beds in mental hospitals (per 100 000 population) [Internet]. WHO. [cited 2018 Oct 2]. Available from: http://www.who.int/gho/mental_health/care_delivery/beds_hospitals/en/

20. Los Angeles Sheriff's Department mental health count. Facilitated by Joseph Ortego, Chief Psychiatrist, Correctional Health Services. Men's Central Jail, Twin Towers Mental Health Unit, Los Angeles: Data Report; March 14, 2018.

21. Los Angeles County Sheriff's Department. Custody division year end review 2016. Los Angeles: Los Angeles County Sheriff's Department;2017.

22. Katz M. Letter to LAC Board of Supervisors from Director of LAC Health Agency: Examination of increase in mental competency cases. September 19, 2016.

23. Churchill LR, Estroff SE, Henderson GE, King NMP, Oberlander J, Strauss R. The social medicine reader, vol. 1–2. 2nd ed. Durham: Duke University Press.

Teaching Population Health and Community Health Assessment to Undergraduate Medical Students

Pyser S. Edelsack, Talha Khan, and Jack Geiger

The Problem

During recent decades, many medical schools and residency programs have tried new curricular approaches to issues of population health, community health status, and the social determinants of health [1–10]. Over the past 40 years, a constantly evolving core curricular effort to achieve these aims has played a central role in teaching at our school. Such efforts have had special relevance at the Sophie Davis School of Biomedical Education (SDBME), with its explicit commitment to two related missions: to expand the pool of underrepresented minorities in medicine and to train primary care physicians for practice in underserved communities. In this paper we describe the current form of an intensive pair of linked courses in community health assessment and direct field placement, designed to meet this educational need.

The SDBME at the City College of New York, located in Central Harlem, is a 7-year BS/MD program. Students, admitted after graduation from high school, spend 5 years at SDBME, during which they complete the first 2 years of the traditional medical school curriculum. They then complete years 3 and 4 of medical school and receive their MD degrees from one of seven traditional participating medical schools in New York and Pennsylvania. As a condition of admission to SDBME, students sign a contract to practice primary care in underserved areas of New York State for at least 2 years after a primary care residency, thus fulfilling an important component of our mission.

P. S. Edelsack · T. Khan
Sophie Davis School of Biomedical Education, City University of New York Medical School, New York, NY, USA

J. Geiger (✉)
Department of Community Health and Social Medicine, Sophie Davis School of Biomedical Education, City University of New York Medical School, New York, NY, USA
e-mail: jgeiger@igc.org

© Springer Nature Switzerland AG 2019
H. Hansen, J. M. Metzl (eds.), *Structural Competency in Mental Health and Medicine*,
https://doi.org/10.1007/978-3-030-10525-9_7

Since its inception in 1973, our program has been successful in its efforts to recruit qualified underrepresented minority students from public and private high schools in New York State, with a focus on New York City and suburban Nassau County. Working with the high school population allows us to identify and support highly motivated students whose ability to meet the challenges of medical school might not be recognized in a traditional premed program. When students come to SDBME, they can identify themselves as medical students on a pathway to the MD degree. By providing heavily subsidized tuition, we attempt to overcome the barriers of limited financial means and poverty of aspiration [11]. Many of our students have been the first in their families to attend college, let alone medical school. Over the years, SDBME has had increasing success enrolling underrepresented minorities (URM), from 19% of the entering class in the early years to 60% in 2012 [12, 13]. Since minority of physicians frequently return to practice in their own communities, increasing their numbers is an important component of improving healthcare in underserved areas [14–18].

Theoretical Framework

Preclinical Training in Community-Oriented Primary Care

In our ongoing attempts to provide students with the skills and understanding they will need for effective practice of primary care in profoundly disadvantaged and disease-burdened communities, the curriculum of the Department of Community Health and Social Medicine (CHASM) has included two intensive community-based experiences. The first, "Practicum in Community Health Assessment," is designed to give students descriptive and analytic skills to understand population health. The second, "Fieldwork in Community Medicine," is a nonclinical clerkship in a healthcare or social service agency that emphasizes how social, economic, environmental, and psychological factors influence the health of individuals, families, and communities. These are followed by other required CHASM courses in epidemiology, health policy, and the US healthcare system and the contribution of the social sciences to the practice of medicine.

To teach community health and its determinants to students in a way that is analogous to their future clinical approach to individual patients, we have adopted the model called community-oriented primary care (COPC), first elaborated by Drs. Sidney and Emily Kark and their colleagues in South Africa in the 1940s [3, 19–24]. The relationship between individual clinical practice and COPC is summarized in Table 1.

The practitioner of COPC seeks answers to the following cardinal questions [19]:

- What is the state of health of the community?
- What are the factors responsible for this state of health?

Table 1 Summary of the complementary functions of clinical and epidemiologic skills in the development of community-oriented primary care

Clinical (Individual in the examination room)	Epidemiologic (Available data and research on population health and the evidence that demonstrates areas in which health status of a population can be improved)
Examination of the patient	Community health assessment
Diagnosis	Community diagnosis
Treatment	Community intervention
Continuing observation	Surveillance of health status and evaluation of interventions

- What is being done in the community about the state of health by the health service system and by the community?
- What more can be done, what is proposed, and what is the expected outcome?
- What measures are needed to continue health surveillance of the community and to evaluate the effects of what is being done?

The course content and teaching methods have been shaped by student evaluations and insights provided by our peer teaching assistants. Over time, these evaluations suggested that our students were not uniformly receptive to what they sometimes perceived as political discussions of healthcare policy; rather, they wanted to learn the specific skills, data sources, and analytic techniques that would enable them to answer the five cardinal questions of COPC for the communities in which they would be practicing in the future. The following sections describe the content and teaching methods currently used in the two courses that prepare students for the practice of COPC in the US healthcare environment.

The Path

Practicum in Community Health Assessment (CHA)

The CHA course is taught in the second year. It serves to give students an initial experience in the analysis of the demographic, socioeconomic, and health status of a defined community. The emphasis is on data related to health disparities and the social determinants of health. The CHA is organized into five main sections: History and Physical Examination, Demography, Socioeconomic Status, Health Indices, and Health Concerns. The students use the key questions of COPC to guide an assessment of their own communities of residence, defined by zip code. Most of our students are still living in their parental homes, so these are communities with which they are familiar. The implicit message is that these analyses and skills are applicable to *all communities*, not just those that are underserved and burdened with disease.

◆ 1847	**City College** founded
◆ 1904–1906	Interborough Rapid Transit (IRT)-the first official **subway** company in NYC- opens, operating from City Hall to 145th St and Broadway.[1]
◆ 1920–1930s	**Harlem Renaissance** increased black population, especially affluent blacks in Hamilton Heights.[2]
◆ 1930–early 1960	**Immigration** of Eastern European, Greek, Cuban, Puerto Rican, and Dominican populations.[3]
◆ 1920–1930s	**"White flight"** peaks–decline in white non-Hispanic population.[4]
◆ Mid–1980s	**Crack epidemic.** Murder rates in I/WH increased by 115% and the number of assaults and arrests were more than twice that of New York City.[5]
◆ 1993-1998	**Crime decreased** drastically: 50% in the 33rd Precinct and 70% in the 34th Precinct.[6]
◆ Early 1990s–present	**Gentrification** of Washington Heights, Hamilton Heights, and Inwood.[7]

Fig. 1 Example of student timeline for a community in New York City. Inwood/Washington Heights (I/WH) Timeline

The History and Physical Examination section of the CHA answers the question: *Why does my community look the way it does today?* This addresses major events or trends that have affected the community. Students develop a timeline and tables that present changes in the population over the past 20–30 years or more, with emphasis on changes in race/ethnicity, immigration, age, gender, language, and socioeconomic status. Each student prepares a map based on his or her direct "shoe leather" observations of the community that includes housing (type and condition), open spaces and institutions, public transportation, and commercial areas (wholesale, retail, or industrial). Figure 1 provides an example of a student's timeline for a community in New York City.

The Demography section of the CHA presents a more detailed description of population variables. Using Infoshare, a free online software package that integrates US Census data and health data by geographic area in New York City and New York State [25], the student examines in greater depth the current structure of the population. Using McFalls' "Population: A Lively Introduction," [26] a useful demographic primer, the students answer the following questions: Is it an old community or young? Is the age and gender structure of the community changing? Is the community growing? Are there identifiable subpopulations that might have special health and social service needs? Each student is required to create an age pyramid of his or her community and to calculate demographic rates, such as change in population over time (the rate of increase or decrease), proportions of the community affected by linguistic isolation, and the age dependency ratio. Students are assigned readings that identify the extent to which such factors are associated with health problems that may be present in their communities.

In the Socioeconomic Status (SES) section, students utilize US Census data to describe occupation, education, and income in their communities. They then refer to relevant articles identifying the extent to which such factors could be associated with the health status of their communities. Each of these SES variables can be examined by race, ethnicity, and gender. Students are also required to create a table showing the social stratification in their communities. Figure 2 is an example of a student's original social stratification table for a community in New York City.

The Health Indices section provides a description and assessment of the key health status indicators, focusing on those that can be improved at the population level. Students use the following data: births and birth outcomes, mortality and morbidity statistics (reportable diseases, hospitalizations), risk factors for disease (Behavioral Risk Factor Surveillance System [BRFSS]), and sentinel events. Students compare their findings to the national goals presented in the federal government's 10-year "Healthy People" targets [27]. Figure 3 is an example of a student's work describing the leading causes of death for a community in New York City, as compared to the national goals.

Social stratification (I/WH: 2006-10)
Source*: American Community Survery, Census Bureau, US Commerce Dept
Source.

Class	Approximate percentage of population	Range of family income
Wel-0ff	2.53%	Greater than $200,000
Upper middle class	9.84%	$100,000 to $199,999
Middle middle class	29.08%	$45,000 to 99,999
Lower middle class	21.61%	$25,000 to $44,999
Poor	36.93%	Less than $25,000

Sources*:

- Rose, stephen. Social Stratification in the United States. The New Press, New York, NY 2007
- Gibert, D. (2002) The American Class Structure: In An Age of Growing Inequality. Belmont, CA: Wadsworth; Thompson, W. & Hickey, J. (2005).
- Society in Focus. Boston, MA: Pearson, Allyn & Bacon; Beeghley, L (2004).
- The Structure of Social Stratification in the United States. Boston, MA; Pearson, Allyn & Bacon.
- The Upper middle class may also be referred to as *Professional class* Ehrenreich, B.(1989). The inner Life of the Middle Class. NY, NY; Harper-Colins.
- Francis, D. Where Do you Fall in the American Economic class system, US News, 2012. Available at http://money. usnews.com/money/personal-finance/articles/2012/09/13/where-do-you-fall-in-the -american-economic-cless-system.

Fig. 2 Example of student social stratification table for a community in New York City

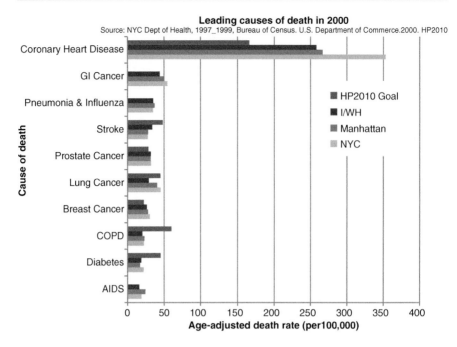

Fig. 3 Example of a student's work describing the leading causes of death for a community in New York City, as compared to the national goals

Students also perform the calculations to determine if their communities qualify as a Medically Underserved Area (MUA) or a Health Professional Shortage Area (HPSA). They explore the available BRFSS data and compare their community's age-adjusted rates to those in other areas and, where applicable, to *Healthy People* goals. Students summarize birth outcome data using infant mortality rates, low birth weight, and the relevant SES variables, such as the mother's education, insurance coverage, race, and ethnicity. They calculate years of potential life lost (YPLL) and identify selected causes of death such as homicide, suicide, and HIV infections. Figure 4 is an example of a student's examination of the leading causes of death by YPLL for a community in New York City.

In the final section, Health Concerns, the students use the data they have gathered and the analyses they have made to identity major health problems such as coronary heart disease, colorectal cancer, etc. and construct a "case for action" that proposes specific interventions to address these problems. In addition, students select one or two subpopulations (e.g., baby boomers, populations living below the poverty line, etc.) at risk for disparate health outcomes. To justify these choices of population groups and health problems, students must cite epidemiologic and other relevant studies in the healthcare literature. The student's case for action must be based on the recommendations of the US Preventive Task Force and community-level interventions promoted by the Centers for Disease Control and Prevention (CDC) and the New York City and State Departments of Health.

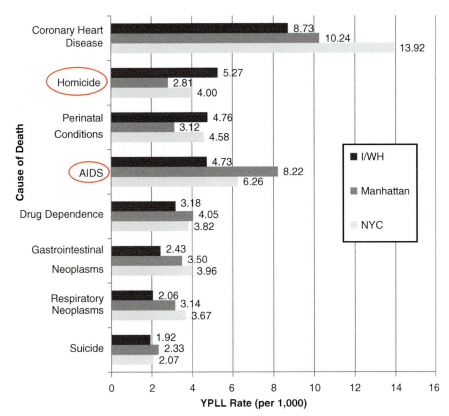

Fig. 4 Example of a student's examination of the leading causes of death by YPLL for a community in New York City

In a second community health assessment exercise, all students, now assigned to small workshop groups, undertake a study of a community of relative poverty in New York City. For this new community setting, they repeat the explorations and analyses that they have performed on their own communities of residence, as described above. There are five workshops, one for each section of the CHA. In each such section, five to seven students are given the relevant data set for that workshop, as well as questions and relevant readings. The final or summative question for each workshop asks the students what additional data are needed to better understand this component of the community health assessment. The research and writing necessary to complete the CHA is a semester-long process that requires time management and continuing reflection and revision. The final papers run 30–50 pages and include all the supporting charts and tables.

This training of students in community health assessment was originally presented as a required lecture series with small group discussion. In 2000, two major changes were implemented. First, a problem-based learning model was introduced, replacing most lectures. Second, each year six students who had done outstanding work in the course in the previous year were selected as teaching assistants (TAs) for the next year's course. Each TA is responsible for facilitating two groups of students in separate workshops.

The selected TAs meet during several months before the start of the CHA course to revise the content and create new materials based on their own experience in the course, student feedback, and the previous year's weekly evaluations. TAs are responsible for creating new data sets for the workshop case study, revising workshop content and the question set for each workshop, and preparing teaching guides used by each TA. A meeting with faculty precedes each week of teaching. This iterative process every year with new TAs has added many new components and methods to our teaching. The TAs perform all this work while continuing their studies in the third-year SDBSE curriculum.

Fieldwork in Community Medicine

After the successful completion of the CHA in the spring of the second year, students begin their first clerkship, "Fieldwork in Community Medicine," during the summer between the second and third years. Students work 20 h a week for 8 weeks in a health or social service agency, interacting with patients and professionals in a community setting. In addition, students conduct a survey and/or chart review defined by their field site for 10–13 h a week. This community-based service and learning experience exposes the students to health and social services and the problems they deal within an underserved, low-income, and high-need community, thus deepening their understanding of the social determinants of health. Students provide navigation assistance, health education, and other services to multiple patients under the supervision of appropriate professional staff, including medical assistants, social workers, public health nurses, community outreach workers, and physicians. This firsthand work experience allows students to gain knowledge of the scope and diversity of patients' problems, as well as of community resources and how they relate, or fail to relate, to the needs of patients. At their fieldwork site, each student completes a survey or clinical chart review aimed at exploring a question defined by the host agency; all data collected belongs to the clerkship site. Students design a questionnaire or data collection form, submit it for agency approval, pilot test it, and make revisions. Students then determine the sample size and selection procedure, describe the limits of the sample, collect and code the data from the target population or selected clinical charts, enter the data into SPSS, and analyze the data. Then the students present their findings at a staff meeting. Near the end of the course, students similarly present a case study of a selected patient they have interviewed in depth. They include such elements as presenting problem, need for social service, health education, behavior modification, wellness plan, and prognosis.

The fieldwork faculty and the agency preceptor evaluate students twice during the summer, as to their professionalism (respect and empathy in interactions with patients), accountability (appropriate utilization of supervision to solve problems), advocacy (assist patients in obtaining services and resources for health and social needs), and verbal and written communication skills, and students are given feedback on their overall performance.

Key Learnings

The combination of training in community health assessment and fieldwork in community medicine is designed to prepare our students for future practice in underserved communities. Our students are assigned their first "patients"—first their own community of residence and then a second community of relative poverty—to determine the potential for improving the health of the entire population, not just patients who come for treatment in a health center. Then in their first clerkship, they see a community from the patient's point of view in the role of advocate and educator.

These courses provide for the acquisition and use of specific skills and methodologies that can be applied in the future by graduating practitioners in underserved areas. The courses are designed not to lecture students about the relationships of social, economic, and environmental factors to community and population health status; rather, they are intended to facilitate a process in which students discover them through their work in these courses. Both of these courses have consistently received extremely high student evaluation ratings. Frequent feedback to us from graduates now practicing in underserved populations indicates that many do indeed remember and apply the skills they learned during these courses and that they continue to influence their modes of practice.

As we have noted, the last few decades have seen ongoing efforts in medical education to achieve these goals by constructing courses to equip medical students with the skills we have described. Such attempts have increasing significance for the future, as major shifts in the demographic composition of the US population loom. We are on the cusp of becoming a "majority minority" population, with increasing proportions of African American, Hispanic, and Asian residents, with proportions of whites remaining significant. At the same time, high prevalence of poverty, and especially urban concentrations of poverty, seems likely to continue. Primary care physicians of the future thus will have increased needs for familiarity with this diversity and for an understanding of the social determinants of health if they are to make significant contributions to the improvement of population health. Further development and continual evolution of courses similar to those we have described may, therefore, be essential to our teaching of medical students now and in the future.

References

1. Sass P, Edelsack P. Teaching community health assessment skills in a problem-based format. Acad Med. 2001;76(1):88–91.
2. Westerhaus M, Finnegan A, Haidar M, Kleinman A, Mukherjee J, Farmer P. The necessity of social medicine in medical education. Acad Med. 2015;90(5):565–8.
3. Mullan F, Epstein L. Community-oriented primary care: new relevance in a changing world. Am J Public Health. 2002;92(11):1748–55.
4. Maeshiro R, Evans CH, Stanley JM, et al. Using the clinical prevention and population health curriculum framework to encourage curricular change. Am J Prev Med. 2011;40(2):232–44.
5. Valentine-Maher SK, Van Dyk EJ, Aktan NM, Bliss JB. Teaching population health and community-based care across diverse clinical experiences: integration of conceptual pillars and constructivist learning. J Nurs Educ. 2014;53(3):S11–8. https://doi.org/10.3928/01484834-20140217-01.
6. Sava S, Armitage K, Kaufman A. It's time to integrate public health into medical education and clinical care. J Public Health Manag Pract. 2013;19(3):197–8. https://doi.org/10.1097/PHH.0b013e3182847b11.
7. Geppert CM, Arndell CL, Clithero A, et al. Reuniting public health and medicine: The University of New Mexico School of Medicine Public Health Certificate. Am J Prev Med. 2011;41(4 Suppl 3):S214–9. https://doi.org/10.1016/j.amepre.2011.06.001.
8. Muller D, Meah Y, Griffith J, et al. The role of social and community service in medical education: the next 100 years. Acad Med. 2010;85(2):302–9. https://doi.org/10.1097/ACM.0b013e3181c88434.
9. Régo PM, Dick ML. Teaching and learning population and preventive health: challenges for modern medical curricula. Med Educ. 2005;39(2):202–13. https://doi.org/10.1111/j.1365-2929.2004.02058.x.
10. Kumpusalo E, Tuomilehto J. Teaching of primary health care in practice: a model using local health centres in undergraduate medical education. Med Educ. 1987;21(5):432–40. https://doi.org/10.1111/j.1365-2923.1987.tb00392.x.
11. Geiger HJ. Sophie Davis School of Biomedical Education at City College of New York prepares primary care physicians for practice in underserved inner-city areas. Public Health Rep. 1980;95(1):32–7.
12. The Sophie Davis School of Biomedical Education Office of Admissions. The incoming classes of 2012 and 2013. The Sophie Davis School of Biomedical Education/CUNY Medical School: 2013.
13. Roman SA. Addressing the urban pipeline challenge for the physician workforce: the Sophie Davis model. Acad Med. 2004;79(12):1175–83.
14. The Center for Health Care Strategies, Robert Wood Johnson Foundation. Advancing primary care: opportunities to support care delivery redesign in practices serving Medicaid and racially and ethnically diverse patients. http://www.rwjf.org/content/dam/farm/reports/reports/2012/rwjf400386. Published August 2012. Accessed 19 Sept 2013.
15. Kirch DG, Nivet M. Increasing diversity and inclusion in medical school to improve the health of all. J Healthc Manag. 2013;58(5):311–3.
16. Castillo-Page L. Diversity in medical education: facts and figures 2012. Washington, DC: Association of American Medical Colleges. https://members.aamc.org/eweb/upload/Diversity%20in%20Medical%20Education_Facts%20and%20Figures%202012.pdf. Published Fall 2012. Accessed 19 Sept 2013.
17. Mullan F, Chen C, Petterson S, Kolsky G, Spagnola M. The social mission of medical education: ranking the schools. Ann Intern Med. 2010;152(12):804–11.
18. The Sophie Davis School of Biomedical Education of the City College of New York. The Sophie Davis Career Outcomes Study. The Sophie Davis School of Biomedical Education/CUNY Medical School: 1998.
19. Kark SL. The practice of community-oriented primary health care. New York: Appleton-Century-Crofts; 1981.

20. Geiger HJ. Community-oriented primary care: the legacy of Sidney Kark. Am J Public Health. 1993;83(7):946–7.
21. Geiger HJ. Community-oriented primary care: a path to community development. Am J Public Health. 2002;92(11):1713–6.
22. Geiger HJ. The meaning of community oriented primary care in the American context. In: Connor E, Mullan F, editors. Community oriented primary care: new directions for health services delivery. Washington, DC: National Academies Press; 1983. p. 60–103.
23. Susser M. Pioneering community-oriented primary care. Bull World Health Organ. 1999;77(5):36–438.
24. Kark SL, Kark E. An alternative strategy in community health care: community-oriented primary health care. Isr J Med Sci. 1983;19(8):707–13.
25. Infoshare Online. http://www.infoshare.org/main/public.aspx. Accessed 15 Sept 2013.
26. McFalls JA. Population: a lively introduction, 5th ed. Popul Ref Bur 2007;62(1) 1–33.
27. Office of Disease Prevention and Health Promotion, U.S. Department of Health and Human Services. www.healthypeople.gov. Accessed 19 Sept 2013.

Part II

Structural Competency in Non-health Sector Collaborations

Urbanism Is a Participatory Sport: Reflections on Teaching About Cities in a School of Public Health

Molly Rose Kaufman, Lourdes Rodriguez,
Robert E. Fullilove III, and Mindy Thompson Fullilove

Our Challenge

The challenge we authors of this case faced was that of learning how to teach urbanism, the science of cities, to students in the Columbia University Mailman School of Public Health. There were several steps in the process. We, ourselves, had to learn to be urbanists. We had to win support for this systems approach. Then we had to develop teaching tools that could work in the context of public health training.

We were all members of a research team—the Community Research Group of New York State Psychiatric Institute and Columbia University—that conducted public health research from 1990 to 2008 in Harlem and other inner-city communities. During our fieldwork, it was impossible to miss the setting or the struggles that accompanied a series of terrible epidemics. People were living in neighborhoods that looked like the aftermath of the apocalypse, filled with boarded-up buildings, vacant lots, illegally dumped trash, and people who suffered from the threat of their surroundings at all times (Fig. 1). What was also clear was that the popular targeted public health programs failed to address the scale and the context of the problems, which were the real sources of ill health. Indeed, these structural processes were often, literally, ruled "out-of-bounds" for public health conversations. It was

M. R. Kaufman
University of Orange, Orange, NJ, USA

L. Rodriguez
Center for Place-Based Initiatives, Dell Medical School, Austin, TX, USA

University of Austin, Texas, Austin, TX, USA

R. E. Fullilove III
Mailman School of Public Health, Columbia University, New York, NY, USA

M. T. Fullilove (✉)
The New School, New York, NY, USA
e-mail: fullilom@newschool.edu

© Springer Nature Switzerland AG 2019   101
H. Hansen, J. M. Metzl (eds.), *Structural Competency in Mental Health and Medicine*,
https://doi.org/10.1007/978-3-030-10525-9_8

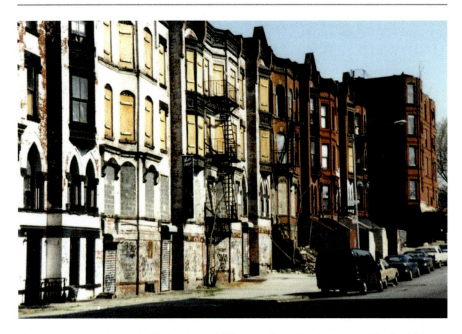

Fig. 1 Boarded-up houses in Harlem in the 1990s were the setting for many epidemics. This setting was not addressed by the standard public health interventions. [With permission from Mindy Fullilove]

common for leaders of programs to say, "We can't do anything about [name a structural factor] so therefore we'll focus on specific, actionable items."

We didn't agree with that argument, but we had to admit we didn't have a better idea. Happily, at a 1993 conference in Paris entitled AIDS, homelessness, and substance abuse, one of us (Mindy Fullilove) met the French urbanist, Michel Cantal-Dupart. In the opening address to the conference, Cantal-Dupart asserted that, when there were serious problems in neighborhoods, the answer was to be found in the organization of the city. He became a mentor to the Community Research Group. We traveled with him to see interventions in many parts of France. He also came to the USA to work with us on projects in Pittsburgh, New York City, and Orange, NJ. Through our visits, assigned readings, and collaboration on projects, Cantal-Dupart trained us to be urbanists and to apply urbanism to the solution of public health problems.

During one of our visits with Cantal-Dupart, we learned about a project to create urbanism training at *Le Conservatoire national des arts et métiers* in Paris (the National Conservatory of Arts and Trades), an important French institution of higher learning that is dedicated to disseminating practical, technical knowledge from subject matter experts in a wide variety of fields. Its faculty was engaged in the practice of their professions, and they shared their expertise with their students. Cantal-Dupart argued that, given that many disciplines cooperated to make great cities, students from many kinds of professional backgrounds should study urbanism together. A department of urbanism—*Urbanism et l'environment*—was created at CNAM, and Cantal-Dupart became its first chair.

We were impressed by the breadth of this vision. It made sense to us that public health students should be among those prepared to engage with the city. We decided that we would develop a program for teaching urbanism. At that time, the School of Public Health had a "track" system. Our proposal to start an urbanism track was accepted and we admitted our first students in 2004.

Our Theoretical Framework

We derived our pedagogy from the ways in which Cantal-Dupart had taught all of us. His urbanism was concerned with the concept that *fracture* was the great injury of the city. Cities function best when their neighborhoods and their commercial centers form an organic whole. When urban centers become divided along race, social class, language, and other demarcating features, what was whole now becomes sundered and fractured. In response, Cantal-Dupart's efforts were directed at identifying the injuries to movement and interaction and repairing them. In order to help us understand this work, he would give us reading assignments and encourage us to study maps and history, and then he would take us to see sights, explain what we were seeing as we walked around, and give us simple diagrams of the places that helped us get the Big Picture. With his unique pedagogical flair, he demonstrated both the problem and the solution in this manner.

During travels with him in 2000, Mindy Fullilove and Robert Fullilove had the opportunity to visit the spectacular chateau and gardens at Vaux-le-Vicomte. Cantal-Dupart demonstrated the ways in which André Le Nôtre had used perspective in the garden. While walking around the beautiful grounds, Cantal-Dupart would stop at vantage points and demonstrate the vistas. It included many surprises. From the chateau, we could see a statue of Hercules in the distance. It looked as if we could walk straight there. But as we walked toward that spot, a canal became apparent, cutting across the garden. We would have had to make a long detour to get to Hercules, but, surprisingly, that canal was completely invisible from the chateau. The miracle of perspective and the numerous ways in Le Nôtre delighted the eyes and the spirit with such varied views of the landscape were memorable. Cantal-Dupart left us with the book, *Un Homme Heureux*, which told us about the life of the designer, the acknowledged founder of the French school of landscape design.

Later that summer, Cantal-Dupart took Mindy and Robert to see a school for prison guards in the city of Agen. He had designed the school's grounds using the techniques of perspective that were demonstrated by André Le Nôtre to create similar vistas and visual delights. We were able to appreciate the application of the idea and its meaning for challenging social fracture. The school, after all, was designed to train correction officers how to maintain a facility for keeping people locked up and confined, but the training offered to these officers would take place in a facility that was open and full of sights to delight the eye. The contrast between the facility that trained them and the facilities in which they would work was important and one that Cantal-Dupart believed would assist the school's students to keep an open mind, a perspective on freedom and confinement that would serve them in the discharge of their duties.

With this model in mind, we developed our program by combining coursework with community engagement. Our coursework revolved around two required courses: urban space and health, taught by Mindy Fullilove, and emerging issues in urbanism, a seminar taught on a rotating basis by Robert Fullilove, Mindy Fullilove, and Lourdes Rodriguez. Students took "selectives"—choosing among a group of courses related to the city—to round out the track requirements. They also had the freedom to take electives throughout the university, which was a rich source for urban history, sociology, planning, and other urban studies.

The heart of our community engagement was one of our projects, influenced by Cantal-Dupart's teaching, City Life Is Moving Bodies (CLIMB). CLIMB had a flexible framework that welcomed student participation while protecting the author-ity of the community groups that led the effort. We also used neighborhood tours, which put into perspective the clinical and epidemiological description of the area and its residents, and walking meetings with community organizers, which chal-lenged the perception of helplessness of the people we sought to serve and instead espoused the idea of neighbors as collaborators. We rounded out the training with special initiatives, trips, and conferences to supplement what our students were learning in the classroom (Fig. 2). We expected those in our track to do a practicum related to urbanism and to write a thesis that drew on what they had seen and read.

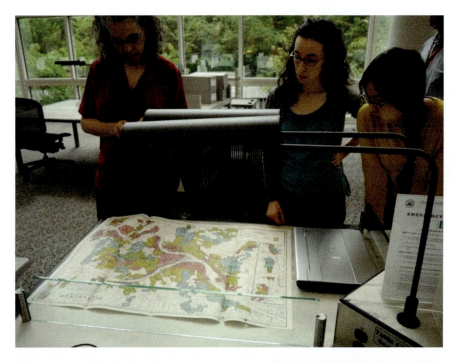

Fig. 2 Mindy Fullilove with urbanism students Samantha Hillson and Amy Yang, at the National Archives at College Park, looking at the redlining map of Pittsburgh. Redlining, instituted by the federal government in 1937, was a major source of urban fracture. [With permission from Mindy Fullilove]

Our Path

The urbanism track was one of the first efforts to bring teaching about the built environment into a school of public health. Our first challenge was completely unexpected. We called our track "Urbanism and Community Health." We soon learned that "community health" was interpreted by public health students to mean "working in a health center in a minority community." We attracted students who wished to be of service to the poor in ways that were fairly traditional in schools of public health. The problem, however, was that they were not interested in cities. The school's track director recognized that we were caught in a clash of expectations and wisely advised that we change the name. "Urbanism and the Built Environment," our new title, spoke to exactly the group we'd hoped to reach, viz., people devoted to cities and committed to making them work for all. We believe that it is useful to start with those whose thinking is closely aligned. We hoped they would provide a bridge to other students, and that proved to be the case.

The second challenge had to do with the school's attitude toward the surrounding neighborhood, a challenge our students took on. Having learned the principles of fracture and its repair in urban settings, our students became actors, helping to challenge the ways in which the school of public health itself perpetuated fracture. They noticed, for example, that the safety officers who spoke during new student orientation advised against crossing Broadway into the Dominican neighborhood in which our offices were located and against walking on the sidewalk that bordered a homeless shelter. The urbanism students challenged this by organizing a neighborhood tour of Washington Heights that took students to many of the community's most important settings. Supported by Professors Bruce Link and Jo Phelan, the urbanism students were able to provide refreshments at a Colonial-era mansion which was the destination for the walk and which provided participants with a much more varied and rich experience of life in one of Manhattan's oldest neighborhoods. This student-led event was institutionalized (and thus sustained over time) when it became part of the formal schedule of activities during orientation week for new graduate students.

Urbanism students worked to name and frame other parts of the town-gown relationship. Columbia University historically was not an ally of the neighboring communities but rather a usurper, slowly incorporating neighborhood land into its domain. The appropriation of Manhattanville to extend the university's main campus was a major land seizure, in which the university used the powers of the state to get land for new buildings. They touted this as "Progress," but refused to answer the question, "Progress for whom?" Our students engaged with these issues in many ways, at one point using the image of a prominent medical center banner—"Amazing things are happening here"—to challenge the dominant narrative in an art exhibit. Their efforts stand as one of the few sustained critiques of the university's neighborhood expansion during a period when many institutions of higher education in the USA were gobbling up land in the name of progress and institutional advancement.

The third challenge was to tackle the public health silos. Problems were typically constructed in tight bundles, such as "adolescent health," "violence prevention," "homelessness," and "food security." It was not easy for the non-urbanism students in Mindy Fullilove's Urban Space and Health class to see the bigger picture. Students in the urbanism track played an important role in class, because they had a more solid understanding of the structural issues of neighborhood inequality that influenced many of the problems. Their contributions to the class discourse around issues of fracture and displacement were invaluable. They could act as intermediaries, using examples from the daily life of students to bridge the gap. They could use the easy examples, like the prohibition on walking by the homeless shelter, to illuminate fracture in the neighborhood. Because these were shared experiences, the urbanism students could help everyone see the larger issues.

Finally, the pedagogy derived from Cantal-Dupart involved sending students into the neighborhood, which is not a simple process. Students arrive at school with preconceptions that echo social movements of the time. These preconceptions color what students think they see. Absent a critical analysis and actively challenging (mis)perceptions, excursions into a neighborhood can lead to the reinforcement of bad information.

Fortunately, with Cantal-Dupart's advice, our team had developed CLIMB. The goal of CLIMB was physical, social, and civic activation of the Northern Manhattan, with a focus on creating a hiking trail to join cliffside parks in Morningside Heights, Harlem, Washington Heights, and Inwood. CLIMB was led by a neighborhood consensus group that made decisions in regular meetings, facilitated by Dr. Lourdes Rodriguez. Students could participate in the consensus group and even take on leadership of our signature annual event, Hike the Heights, a one-day group walking tour of the cliffside parks in Northern Manhattan, without disturbing the careful processing that the group followed. Our CLIMB project offered an excellent setting for student engagement. They were helpers, not leaders, and they were supporting the work of local organizations. That role allowed them to build their community organizing muscles and strengthen their capacity for humility.

For students, it is essential to provide a value-centered context and a robust partnership, as otherwise their prejudices and preconceptions can take over the leadership of the project. This is never helpful. A strong project, by contrast, shifts the way participants think about and treat the neighborhood, bringing them into a right relationship with the vulnerable entity. In this way, they become part of the solution, and not part of the problem. Indeed, inside the protected space of partnership, their particular insights and talents can become powerful contributors to making a better city.

The Key Learning

We believe that seeing change over time is the heart of great urbanism pedagogy and what we aspired to provide our students. Numerous urbanism students wrote essays for a book about the CLIMB project. Ken Nadolski wrote:

Dr. Mindy Fullilove taught me that our cities are fractured and we must work to restore the connections that strengthen the urban fabric in order to improve health. CLIMB's mission has been to increase the physical, social, and civic activity in the communities of northern Manhattan through the promotion of an urban hiking trail that connects Fort Tryon Park, Highbridge Park, Jackie Robinson Park, St. Nicholas Park, Morningside Park, and Central Park. In other words, CLIMB is all about making connections. By connecting the parks, the trail also connects neighborhoods and people. It was always exciting to see these connections come to life at the annual Hike the Heights event. [1]

Another student, Sarah Townley, built on the same observation:

Year after year I began to recognize people from meetings, from previous years, and eventually from my own neighborhood. Polite introductory conversations with familiar faces eventually evolved into "ok now how can we best look at this zoning proposal, how can we best understand how gentrification is affecting our neighborhoods, do you want to go to that meeting with me?" Or "how about we meet up on Saturday and clean this space in the park." "Hey I didn't know there was a homeless shelter in the neighborhood…how can I get involved?" And even "how can your school and my school work together for better health opportunities for students in our district?" [2]

This is the heart of what we hoped that they might see and experience. We believe that anyone who has been through a process of change comes to have faith that change is possible. While they might not have all the skills they need to make change, they have the basic belief in change that city-makers need if we are to move from fracture to restoration.

Our urbanism track ended in 2011. While the track ended—and only one of us remains at Mailman as of this writing—we are all engaged in teaching urbanism. More importantly, alumni of the track have gone on to doctoral programs, including medical school, positions in health departments and health philanthropy, and work in community-based organizations that are working to improve the city. They use these principles and apply them in their analysis of situations. In doing so, they are teaching by doing. The core lessons we learned continue to prove powerful:

- It is essential to have people move through the city if they are to begin to understand how policies that lead to exclusion, segregation, and fracture operate in the real world.
- We need to pair readings with hands on change-work that is sustained over time and handed from "generation to generation" (i.e., from one graduating class to the next), since it is in the accumulation of these experiences that we see long-term impact.
- We must insist that fracture can be fixed, but if and only if we recognize its existence. We cannot make ourselves or others responsible for addressing a wrong, absent the awakening that comes from recognition.

How Can This Learning Be Applied in Other Situations?

We learned that public health's siloed interventions had little to offer to devastated inner-city communities. We had to move out from those narrow interventions and become actors in the city. Our accomplishment lies in learning to practice and teach urbanism, the science of urban ecosystems. As healthcare workers come to the limits of biomedicine and learn that they must have structural competence to make new advances, they, too, will come to see the importance of learning about and teaching structures. We couldn't have taught urbanism before learning it ourselves. So our own openness to new methods was critical. Then, once we had begun to teach urbanism, our students almost immediately became actors in the school and in the city. While this was an outcome we desired, we did not anticipate the creativity and speed with which the students moved. In fact, they became powerful forces for improvement. These lessons can be applied in many settings that have reached the limits of individualism and need new tools to create health and manage disease.

References

1. Nadolski K. Making connections and building partnerships. CLIMB Chronicles; 2017 Sep: 83.
2. Townley S. More than just one day. CLIMB Chronicles; 2017 Sep: 78.

Promoting Collective Recovery in an Immigrant/Refugee Community Following Massive Trauma

Jack Saul

The Problem

How do mental health practitioners deal with the collective and individual traumas faced by a large group of refugees following war and forced migration? Can we use a model that takes into consideration the effects on an entire community rather than trying to solve their problems on a case-by-case basis? This case study describes a collaborative project between mental health professionals and Liberian refugees and immigrants in a neighborhood of Staten Island, New York, that supported the participation of residents within and volunteers from outside the community to respond to the complicated tasks of building a life in a new country. Starting with an approach aimed at shoring up the resilience of the community as a whole, the project participants first aimed to promote greater social cohesion and mutual support among community members. But this was not an easy task in a highly fragmented and polarized community where local organizations competed for sparse resources in one of the most underserved neighborhoods of New York City. Each step along the way in this multi-year project required creative problem-solving to address new and unforeseen challenges – from mobilizing participation, to finding ways of making bridges between a suspicious group of immigrants and available resources, to addressing local corruption, and to healing intense conflict between community members, often fueled by the traumas of their recent war experiences.

Here is a case study in which a structurally competent framework can be useful for community engagement. This case study tells the story of how, given limited resources, the project participants responded to the needs of a majority of members of a community while also finding help for those with the greatest difficulties. Despite the many challenges, they were able to promote health and well-being among community members by strengthening social relationships and cooperation,

J. Saul (✉)
International Trauma Studies Program, New York City, NY, USA

© Springer Nature Switzerland AG 2019
H. Hansen, J. M. Metzl (eds.), *Structural Competency in Mental Health and Medicine*,
https://doi.org/10.1007/978-3-030-10525-9_9

supporting members to participate in community life and local community politics, and by increasing their access to a variety of needed resources. What we learned in our work with this community of West African refugees in Staten Island, New York, may be applicable to other such situations around the world.

Background

As a mental health professional, I had worked with communities affected by massive psychosocial trauma in postwar Kosovo, as well as in Lower Manhattan following the 9/11/01 terrorist attacks. Both of these projects mobilized community members to participate in a collective recovery project [1]. My first encounter with members of the Liberian community in Staten Island was on a visit to a youth recreation center run by one of the community leaders. At the time in 2002, the non-profit organization I directed worked together with three other agencies in the New York area to provide psychological, social, legal, and educational services for refugees. We had begun to have conversations about our services with some of the leaders of this West African community – where a few thousand of its members lived in close proximity in a housing project in the neighborhood of Park Hill. While caseworkers and psychotherapists offered clinical services through some of the programs in our consortium, we were acutely aware of the limitations of an exclusively clinical approach to helping those who had endured political violence and were now facing the challenges of a life in exile from their home countries. Seeking mental health services was problematic for many refugees because of its stigma and their unwillingness to turn into an illness the normal distress that was a consequence of having lived through the difficult experiences of war and the loss of life, property, homeland, and culture.

From my experience working with war survivors in Kosovo and responding to the 9/11/01 terrorist attacks in my neighborhood in Lower Manhattan, I had learned that the most effective programs were those that enhanced the existing strengths of families and communities and did not rely solely on importing the specialized services of professionals. By enhancing their capacities to provide mutual support, problem solve, and engage in the search for meaning and purpose following catastrophe, they would be taking advantage of invaluable resources to promote their healing and recovery. Based on this perspective, our team sought a way of addressing the challenges that all members of the Liberian community must have been facing having just fled the civil wars in their country.

Our funding for this project was aimed at providing services for torture survivors. Since a majority of community members experienced some form of torture or abuse at the hands of government or rebel soldiers, it made sense to promote the collective recovery of the entire community. In most cases, we find that funders need to be educated about how to step out of a framework that primarily focuses on the individual's symptom reduction and consider addressing the health and well-being of the community as whole. Fortunately, in this case, the funding criteria were flexible enough to justify such an innovative approach. This form of community engagement, we believed, was important for building the capacity of residents to access services and utilized them effectively.

The Community

Before beginning to work with the Liberian community, we familiarized ourselves through reading and meeting with country experts with the history and culture of Liberians as well as the recent political situation, wars, and migration flows. West African immigrants had immigrated into northern Staten Island in the 1980s. Their numbers increased, especially those of Liberians, who were fleeing the civil wars from 1989 to 2003. This Liberian community was one of the largest on the East Coast of the USA and became a regular stopping point for those traveling between communities from Boston to Philadelphia and further south. Some of the older residents described a vital community of immigrants who regularly congregated under a large tree in Park Hill, where the elders sold the favored Liberian dishes they cooked at home and people gathered to share information and keep up with the news from the home country. Eventually the assembly "under the tree" ended when the tree was cut down to make way for a Home Depot, and the most vibrant community gatherings began to appear in the Liberian churches and mosques.

Liberian immigrants have a particularly unique history in the USA. Liberia as a country was established by freed or freeborn blacks in the USA in 1847 and became the first republic in Africa. It was believed that these freed blacks had a better chance of pursuing their freedom in Africa while reducing the threat of widespread emancipation of slaves in the USA following the civil war. The Americo-Liberians imported their culture to Liberia and became the power holders, preventing the indigenous majority population from both economic and political participation.

The population fleeing the Liberian civil wars consisted of both Americo-Liberians and indigenous Liberians who imported and performed the historical tensions in their new US communities. Common to both groups was an underlying ambivalence toward the USA, especially the Clinton and Bush II administrations who many Liberians felt had a historical obligation to have prevented or at least impeded the conflict that led to the death and displacement of over half million people and destroyed what had been a thriving economy. Before the wars, Liberia had been one of the most economically advanced countries in Africa. The war almost entirely erased that development, destroying the country's infrastructure and institutions. A subtext of American racism is also felt in relation to the unwillingness of the USA to grant most Liberian immigrants full refugee status. This status would lead to citizenship rather than temporary protective status that required regular renewal by congress. Under the current administration, a large part of the Liberian population is currently at risk for deportation in 2019 due a cancellation of their temporary protective status.

It is estimated that approximately two to three thousand Liberian immigrants live within a few blocks of each other in Park Hill and surrounding streets where many were able to have their rents subsidized. According to a survey conducted among community residents, 90% of them arrived during the civil wars and over 70% reported having experienced the violence of the war directly witnessed murders and experienced severe loss or torture. During the wars, many children in the community were unable to attend schools for up to 7 years. The greatest challenge they face was that of educating their children while living in a neighborhood where they were exposed to a high level of communal violence.

African students entering primary and high schools in New York were not only years behind other students; they often faced tensions with African American students who did not understand their culture. Park Hill was quite dangerous, and families feared letting their children move freely in the neighborhood because of the potential for gang- and drug-related violence. The neighborhood often referred to as "Crack Hill" had one of the highest crime rates in the city. Access to resources was hindered by the fact that Staten Island – the borough mainly accessed by ferry – was not so easily accessible by volunteers who wanted to help and made it difficult for Liberian groups across the city to connect and work together.

Our project team which changed over time primarily consisted of myself, a social work supervisor, and two student interns. It is often assumed that groups of people living together make up a coherent community ready to respond to the offers to provide needed services. But there is much variation in the composition of "communities." We quickly learned, as in many refugee and immigrant enclaves, most of the residents did not previously know each other in their home country. In fact it was likely in this group of Liberians that one might find oneself living among those who had been on opposite sides of the civil conflict. Some victims of persecution were shocked to see those who had abused them during the wars walking freely on the streets of their neighborhood. With over 13 tribal groups, most political parties, as well as supporters of the two rival football teams, there were tremendous tensions. One might say that this was a fragmented community at an early stage of formation. In working collaboratively in such situations, it is important to understand the stage of development and to not be pessimistic. The collective traumas of war and migration lead to social fractures, tensions, and conflict and will need to be understood and addressed when working with such a community.

Theoretical Background of Our Approach

One important point of working with immigrants in the structural competency framework is to establish a partnership in addressing the psychosocial challenges they faced. We began with the ideal of establishing a collaboration with members of the Liberian community, but it quickly becomes apparent that as parties begin to work together, this "collaboration" is a complex social process that is itself defined through the developing relationship. Often romanticized, collaboration may easily ignore the asymmetrical power dynamics that exist between the providers and recipients of services. There are many types of cooperative efforts, ranging from those that are provider driven to those are initiated and sustained by community members. The partnerships that may develop in collaborative work may include a variety of ways of sharing work, of establishing priorities, and of deciding who takes the lead at different times in the process of working together. The particular approach we took is based on the LINC model of community resilience developed by Dr. Judith Landau, [2, 3] in which providers engage community members as active participants in the process of addressing community challenges and not as passive recipient of services. Rather than importing models developed elsewhere, our approach is to develop approaches to problems in partnership with the local community through an iterative process, much like a designer testing prototypes with ongoing input from those who will be utilizing the services developed.

The LINC community resilience approach assumes that communities harbor resources that enable them to recover from adversity. The work with communities must begin with invitation, authority, permission, and a commitment from the community. This approach seeks to engage the entire system of the community, including the representation of individuals and subsystems presenting all cultural and ethnic groups, economic, cultural and social status strata, and the natural support systems such as families, faith-based groups, and the ancillary of helping systems. To reach out and invite such a broad representation from the community takes a lot of work from an initial committed group of participants.

Whether the initial meeting consists of community leaders or is a publically run community forum, the goal of such an approach is to bring people together and identify scripts, themes, and patterns across generations and community history. In the case of an immigrant population such as this group of Liberians, it was important to connect with the stories of life in the home country, before and after the wars and migration. Embedded in these stories are the strengths they may use to address the current challenges they face as a community. For example, the social support they derived from the church community and counsel from religious leaders were practices from Liberia that were readily recreated in the USA. Other practices, like a strong family and school collaboration, were more challenging to establish in Staten Island. Once the strengths, resources, and current challenges are identified, they are then prioritized and turned into realistic tasks and practical projects. These tasks and projects, as will be described in the following sections, focused a great deal on addressing the needs of children and youth. In this approach, community members acting as change agents or links become the leaders and intermediaries between the community members and outside service providers. Because community members direct the project themselves, they are more likely to feel ownership of the project and its subsequent successes, thus increasing their sense of collective efficacy [2].

In working with and supporting community links, it is more likely that such a process can be sustained long after the so-called outside experts have run out of funding and departed. Change agents from within are considerably more effective in effecting change because they are often the best judges of what change is possible, they understand the limitations and obstacles that need to be surmounted, and they are aware of available resources and the resources needed from outside. These links are often in the best position to work collaboratively with fellow citizens in developing creative solutions to current problems and to evaluate and determine which factors have the most impact in promoting the desired change. The success of the LINC model is that the community strengthens its capacity to work together, to recognize and access resources, to provide mutual support and hope, and to develop new communal narratives that give the experiences they have been through meaning and purpose [4].

Challenge 1: How Do We Even Begin to Collaborate with a Fragmented Community?

As will often be the case when working with communities from a structural competency framework, we need to be aware of where the community may fall along a continuum that ranges from social cohesion to fragmentation. The initial stage of our work involved reaching out to local leaders, conducting interviews, and implementing a survey about how Liberians were doing in Park Hill and how they could best address mental health and psychosocial needs. We quickly became aware that this was a community that was highly fragmented. To get the process going, we organized a series of meetings in which community leaders simulated role-plays of families illustrating typical problems they were facing. We held mock community meetings with leaders instructing us about the viewpoints of different community actors such as ministers, local organizations, healthcare providers, youth workers, parents, youth, and elders. This process allowed for the main stakeholders to be identified. We learned that there was a great deal of tension between local organizations due to the competition for limited resources. Local funders had given financial support to African-run organizations but ended that support due to problems with accountability. This left the organizations with few options for adequate funding with the largest organization acting as a gatekeeper preventing new groups of immigrants from access to funding.

The solution to this first challenge was to bring together in a consortium the important stakeholders including the Liberian community organizations, churches, refugee resettlement agencies, and other social service providers working with the community. The consortium met monthly at Kortu's, the local Liberian restaurant, to map out community resources, to prioritize community needs, and to develop practical projects to address those needs. The consortium allowed different groups to develop a more collaborative approach and determine how limited resources could be used. The first priority to emerge was how to provide after-school and weekend activities for youth including addressing the needs of unsupervised Liberian youth living on the streets and rooftops in the projects.

Challenge 2: How Does the Consortium Address the Psychosocial Challenges of Youth?

Since there were no organization with the capacity to address youth psychosocial needs at the time, some community members from the consortium offered to set up a Saturday afternoon program for Liberian youth at a church not far from the housing project. The four members that came forth and proposed this program eventually became the community links (community change agents). These members had prior experience running youth programming in Liberia and in the USA. With a very small budget, the Link team organized a program by engaging adults who had an interest or special skill to offer youth. The funding came in handy to provide transportation, lunch, and recreational supplies.

The Link team put together an interesting program combining a rap group taught by Liberian musicians that presented scenarios of effective peer relations, a computer education program, and video history project for teens about their lives in Liberia before immigration. The program was initiated with a forum in which all the 50 program youth gathered to listen to a former Liberian president and community member, David K, speak about his experience during his short interim presidency. Youth asked him questions about the history and culture of Liberia.

In a systems approach to psychosocial programming, much is learned by implementing a small project and learning from observation how the project is received, what works, what needs improvement, and what is the systemic impact on the community. We learned that such a program needed to take place within walking distance of where the youth lived – transportation was a challenge, and parents were not so comfortable with the distance children had to go away from home. We also learned through the consortium and the current project that there was a great deal of talent among adults in the community that could be engaged in future programs. Most important we learned that by supporting a new group in the community working outside the gatekeeper's program was threatening, upset the status quo, and was met with resistance. Our assumption that these activities would be a welcome offering for a community paucity of resources was incorrect. Instead, our efforts initiated a power struggle in the consortium and the community at large that would continue for months afterward.

With limited resources, an ongoing power struggle, the need to bring services geographically closer to families, and the realization of a tremendous resource in enthusiasm and talents of community members, the Link team decided to create their own community organization. It didn't take them long to reach out to the housing project management and receive a donated ground floor apartment they could develop into a community space. This created a momentum that was not hindered by gatekeeper resistance, and quickly the space opened a drop-in center, filled with donated furniture, computers, a TV, and young community members and students who wanted to volunteer their assistance. Three project leaders from the community enlisted, trained, and monitored the work of volunteers.

The project developed a drop-in center in the donated space, which grew organically in response to the stated needs of those coming to the center and the available residents and student volunteers who could help out. A model was developed in which student volunteers were trained to work alongside the local community volunteers to promote psychosocial projects. For instance, one of the initial programs based on such collaboration was cultural group for children which arranged for elders, artists, poets, and musicians from the community to come share what they knew about Liberian culture, arts, and other resources. An example of one project was Coming Home: Connecting Elders in the Diaspora with Family and Friends Back Home [3]. http://www.itspnyc.org/african_refuge/cominghome.html

Challenge 3: Access to Resources

While services were available in Staten Island, Liberian community members weren't leaving their homes to access those services due to lack of trust of outsiders, challenges with transportation, need to help to navigate bureaucratic systems, and challenges with illiteracy. With a foundation established at the drop-in center, its staff earned the trust of residents who saw the value of the initial services they were offering. But bringing more substantial services like casework staff or legal and employment help required more financial resources than were available for a program run by African staff. To meet this challenge, the drop-in center became a bridge between community members and outside provider organizations.

Wagner School of Nursing in Staten Island arranged a practicum for nursing students to provide supervised work on site for residents one day per week. The nursing students would carry out examinations, monitor blood pressure, and help with understanding and managing prescription medications, offering advice on diet and exercise, and referring those who needed more specialized services to a doctor at the mobile health van which began to park in front of the center each week.

While the community's capacity to take advantage of services was being enhanced, larger social service agencies in the surrounding neighborhoods began to receive funding to help African community members with mental health and social services. But community members were not so inclined to leave the housing project and meet with outside organizations. These large organizations looked to the drop-in center staff to make the connections and do their outreach for them, but without compensation for the enormity of work this entailed. One problem is that funders often neglect supporting the kind of capacity building the drop-in center had developed and without support to sustain it – such uncompensated outreach can put a strain on small community organizations.

Once the drop-in center was established, like a garden with fertile soil, all kinds of projects began to spring up: artist's collaboration, cultural programs, street festivals, concerts, and other activities that promote interaction between African immigrants and their African American and Hispanic neighbors. The success of the program led to the donation of a basement space that was renovated by the community and turned into a youth center with a much needed after-school program.

Challenge 4: Supporting Community Cohesion While Challenging the Status Quo

While it appeared there was cohesion within the community, there was a deep, unseen level of competition and conflict between some of the organizations. Much of this was due to our having supported this new group of community actors to create a program that upset the status quo. The team of community links wanted to promote a collaborative approach to solving community problems, but the "links" felt they needed to challenge the existing organization in the community, because they believed that the most powerful organization was exploiting community members. They wanted to expose and challenge this corruption. This ended up polarizing our program.

We were now drawn into the community conflict supporting one faction in the community. We had been working hard to be neutral and promote collaboration among the groups. When one of the leaders of another organization approached me and wanted me to diffuse the conflict, by placing constraints on the people working within the organization we were supporting, this led to a dilemma. To what extent do we give in to this pressure to encourage those in our organization to not participate in the political activity in the community, which they felt to be most needed? Part of our intervention was to support members to engage in civic participation, the political life of the community.

While in the development field, these challenges are expected, recognized, and addressed; it may come as a shock to clinicians and those in the health field, who are often taught to seek neutrality and to avoid engagement in the political context. You will be engaged in the political context and must allow space for communities to shape their civic participation and political voice.

But like families in clinical therapeutic situation, the rigidity to change must be challenged by the therapist rather than support a family maintaining its previous dysfunctional homeostasis. The same holds for communities on the cusp of change, in which there may be need for outside providers to unbalance the system by supporting one side of a conflict. We ended up supporting the community links in advocating for greater transparency and accountability in the Liberian Community Association. They took the lead on taking this position, and by doing so, our collaborative team lost our position of neutrality in the local consortium of service providers.

Challenge 5: Engaging with the Legacy of Conflict in the Home Country and Local Community

Can a people move forward and rebuild their lives while addressing issues of truth and accountability? This question sparked a debate and tension both in Liberia and in the Staten Island Liberian community. Relieved that the war had finally come to an end and democracy was restored, the early aspirations of Liberians were to both move on and reckon with the past. Collective trauma is seen by those who have endured such a catastrophe as a moral challenge. Not only has the physical environment and infrastructure been destroyed, and thousands have been killed and injured, but the social and moral order has been disrupted. Thus, it is the responsibility of the collective to understand the conditions that led to and sustained the conflict, the individuals and institutions that contributed, and to determine how best to prevent such a tragedy in the future.

There were a variety of viewpoints among the Liberian residents of Park Hill. Many felt challenged just to support themselves and their children in New York. They preferred to trust the new government to handle the changes and process of reckoning. Others in the neighborhood felt that effort is needed to be made to examine the recent past and threw their support to the Liberian Truth and Reconciliation Commission. This commission had been established by the Liberian government as a condition for ending the war and was tasked to explore the difficult questions about the war's origins and its course and to bring to light the abuses that took place during the war.

This tension expressed itself most acutely in the debate about what to convey to children, youth, and teenagers about the wars. For example, a debate arose around showing a film called, the Uncivil War, which graphically exposes the history and horrors of the civil war in Liberia. The community addressed this tension by deciding that the film was not appropriate for children under 13. Years later, at a community event, they watched the film, Pray the Devil Back to Hell, which provided a more hopeful outlook on the circumstance that led to the end of the war in Liberia, including the role that women played in promoting peace process. This film was deemed more appropriate for showing to children. Liberian adults wanted their children to know the history of Liberia, its culture, and its hardships but did not want them to have such an adverse reaction to the events depicted in film that they would never want to return with their families to the home country.

Over the next few years, the community created a number of spaces for addressing the experiences of the war as well as discussing holding those who acted most brutally during the war. Many were upset that the greatest criminals of the war were members of the government and financially benefiting themselves in a culture of impunity.

At this time, the tensions between moving on and holding people accountable for past injustices were heightened in the community as the Liberian Truth and Reconciliation Commission began taking statements about war experiences from community members. This TRC was the first to those Liberians displaced to other countries, including the USA. The center's staff as well as other organizations worked together to publicize the fact that local interviewers would take statements.

We were also invited by members of the community to create a theatrical piece based on the testimonies of diverse Liberian voices speaking about their war experiences. This theater piece, performed both inside the community and for the public outside Staten Island, was entitled "Checkpoints" referring to the life-threatening circumstance most Liberians experienced as they were migrating from place to place during the conflict. Checkpoints was later performed in 2010 at an international conference organized by center staff on the Liberian Truth and Reconciliation Commission, which included commissioners and public figures from Liberia. It addressed the findings and recommendations made in the TRC report.

Inspired by the TRC process now taking place in Staten Island as well as Liberia, a ministerial leader, who had returned to the community from Liberia after the war, organized a local reconciliation process between churches, nonprofit groups, and other stakeholders who had been struggling with each other over years. He initiated dialogues to "wipe the slate clean" and recommit to the deeply held Liberian values of community service. The process led to a lessening of tensions and greater cooperation among the local organizations.

The Key Learning

Collective trauma, the shared injuries to a population's social, cultural, and physical ecologies, requires collective responses. It is important not to disregard the ways families and communities harbor remarkable capacities for adaptation after tragedy. As providers, working with a structural competency framework with communities that have suffered from war and forced migration, it is helpful to ally and support those in the community who are committed to addressing the psychosocial needs of their community as whole. As this process unfolds many challenges arise along the way, and the direction the community chooses may not be immediately apparent to outside supporters. The shape of this resilience is culturally based, socially constructed over time, and varies according to circumstances. Community recovery is a relational process and requires creative improvisation. Its success depends on competent leadership and the restoration of caring, trusting relationships.

References

1. Saul J. Collective trauma, collective healing: promoting community resilience in the aftermath of disaster. 1st ed. New York: Routledge; 2013.
2. Landau J. Communities that care for families: the LINC model for enhancing individual, family, and community resilience. Am J Orthopsychiatry. 2010;80(4):516–24.
3. Landau J, Saul J. Facilitating family and community resilience in response to major disaster. In: Walsh F, McGoldrick M, editors. Living beyond loss. New York: Norton; 2004.
4. Fullilove M, Saul J. Rebuilding communities post-disaster: lessons from 9/11. In: Neria Y, Gross R, Marshall R, Susser E, editors. 9/11: mental health in the wake of terrorist attacks. Cambridge: Cambridge University Press; 2004. p. 164–77.

Is Poverty Making Me Sick? An Example of the Impact of Medical-Legal Partnership on Keeping Children Healthy

Andrew F. Beck, Mallory Curran, Adrienne W. Henize, Melissa D. Klein, Donita S. Parrish, Edward G. Paul, and Elizabeth Tobin-Tyler

Abbreviations

CCHMC	Cincinnati Children's Hospital Medical Center
Child HeLP	Cincinnati Child Health-Law Partnership
MLP	Medical-legal partnership
PPCC	Pediatric Primary Care Center
SDH	Social determinants of health

A. F. Beck (✉)
Divisions of General & Community Pediatrics and Hospital Medicine, Cincinnati Children's Hospital Medical Center, Cincinnati, OH, USA

Department of Pediatrics, University of Cincinnati College of Medicine, Cincinnati, OH, USA
e-mail: Andrew.Beck1@cchmc.org

A. W. Henize · M. D. Klein
Division of General and Community Pediatrics, Cincinnati Children's Hospital Medical Center, Cincinnati, OH, USA

M. Curran
Mallory Curran Consulting, Brooklyn, NY, USA

D. S. Parrish
Legal Aid Society of Greater Cincinnati, Cincinnati, OH, USA

E. G. Paul
Department of Family Medicine, St. Joseph's Hospital & Medical Center/Dignity Health, Phoenix, AZ, USA

E. Tobin-Tyler
Department of Family Medicine, Warren Alpert Medical School of Brown University, Providence, RI, USA

Department of Health Services, Policy and Practice, Brown University School of Public Health, Providence, RI, USA

© Springer Nature Switzerland AG 2019   121
H. Hansen, J. M. Metzl (eds.), *Structural Competency in Mental Health and Medicine*,
https://doi.org/10.1007/978-3-030-10525-9_10

SNAP   Supplemental Nutrition Assistance Program
USDA   United States Department of Agriculture
WIC   Special Supplemental Nutrition Program for Women, Infants, and
                Children

Introduction

Physicians who serve vulnerable patient populations often struggle to identify and address risks related to the social determinants of health (SDH). These often complex structural issues and institutional barriers affect patients' health and include risks related to substandard housing and lack of access to basic supports like health insurance and food assistance. Many of these barriers to health have significant legal underpinnings – e.g., enforcement of housing safety ordinances and erroneous delays and denials of eligibility for Medicaid and programs like the Supplemental Nutrition Assistance Program (SNAP). Still, it can be overwhelming and discouraging for physicians as they try to tackle such complex nonclinical issues on their own. Physicians need partners, both inside the clinic and in the community, to effectively address the needs of their patients. The following case study explores the value of the medical-legal partnership (MLP) approach in addressing risks related to the SDH. MLPs embed legal professionals and law students alongside healthcare professionals to address social and structural barriers to patient and population health through training and education, consultation, referral, and collaborative upstream problem-solving [1].

Below, we introduce a clinical case in order to illustrate the ways that MLPs can provide an evidence-based approach to identifying and managing health-relevant social and environmental risks. The case is one that is not uncommon in pediatrics; although similar issues could come up in other practice areas, including family medicine and obstetrics. Specifically, through the case below, we illustrate the value of a systematic approach to SDH screening, referral of appropriate cases to an MLP's legal advocates, and ongoing analysis of population-level patterns that emerge from individual patient cases reviewed by MLPs. We highlight how such strategies ultimately empower clinicians to affect structural changes in ways that can improve the health of their individual patients and their patient panels more broadly.

Section 1: A Common Medical Case

It is a hot day in early summer. You cannot believe it is more than 90° in May. You are thankful for air conditioning, to say the least! You are a 2nd year pediatric resident with a busy schedule, and your first patient just arrived. You look down at your docket for the day only to see the appointment is a "twofer," a brother and sister coming to see you together. The brother is a 7-year-old boy named Chris. He is being seen for a follow-up visit as he was discharged from the hospital 2 days ago. His sister, Brianna, is being seen for a weight check; she is 2 months old with a chief complaint of "poor weight gain." You try to spend your last minute before knocking on their door preparing yourself for the visit. How will you assess their medical risks? Are there other concerns or triggers likely to be raised? How will you respond?

Will this be a quick in-and-out visit, or are you poised to start your day behind? Finally ready, you knock on the door.

You start with Chris. Between your review of the electronic health record and your discussion with him and his mother, Ms. Williams, you uncover the following. Just days ago, Chris was hospitalized for roughly 48 h due to an acute asthma exacerbation. He is a known asthmatic, and this is his third lifetime admission; his second was in the last 6 months. He has also visited the emergency department multiple times for asthma in the last year. During his recent inpatient stay, he was placed on the evidence-based protocol for asthma management and left the hospital feeling better than when he was admitted. He is on two daily controller medications, and Chris and Ms. Williams report that he takes them both "most of the time." On your physical examination, Chris seems to be breathing comfortably. He is not actively wheezing. You are pleased that he seems to have improved from his acute asthma attack.

You move on to his younger sister, Brianna. Prior to entering the room, you had noticed some concerning aspects of her growth curve. She has not been growing at the velocity that you would have liked to have seen. This is also not a new complaint or concern – Brianna was recently seen by a colleague of yours who had been tracking her weight closely. The dietician saw her at the last visit as well. Ms. Williams says that Brianna continues to exclusively breastfeed and does not have any emesis. Ms. Williams is fairly certain she has adequate milk supply; the child latches well and is feeding every 3 h, even at night. Brianna has had the requisite number of wet and dirty diapers. Her physical examination is normal and does not point to any specific organic causes of her poor weight gain.

You leave the room to discuss both of these children with your preceptor. To summarize, you have a 7-year-old boy who has gotten over the worst of an acute asthma exacerbation and a 2-month-old girl who, you are worried, is failing to thrive. For Chris, you are tempted to ensure that he has adequate supply of his acute and chronic asthma medications and plan to see him back in 2–3 months. For Brianna, you are contemplating asking Ms. Williams to fill out a detailed feeding diary to more effectively identify how much Brianna is truly eating. You are then considering a follow-up visit with both in 1 month. Are these plans adequate? Would other, as yet unasked, questions lead you down different paths, ones that could more effectively identify and address common root causes? Can we look at these same cases using a different lens?

Section 2: Shifting Perspective

We frequently fall into heuristics that prompt us to see clinical cases narrowly. As physicians, we may become accustomed to treating certain ailments in certain ways such that we may miss clues that would appropriately take us off that standard path. For example, asthma is generally treated using evidence-based protocols. These protocols help us to effectively manage acute exacerbations or attacks. They may not, however, provide us with the tools to identify triggers of that attack. Such protocols can at times create blinders, streamlining, and/or oversimplifying our approach to problems or issues that may be inherently complex [2]. How can we break free from a mindset that might be limiting our ability to see the forest for the trees (without, of course, ignoring the trees themselves)?

Health inequities in childhood are widespread and are often exacerbated by risks related to the SDH. For example, much is now known about the higher incidence and severity of asthma among children who live in substandard housing [3–5]. Although children living in low-income households are somewhat more likely to be diagnosed with asthma, they are far more likely to suffer the worst outcomes due in large part to adverse environmental exposures [2, 5–7] – they are far more likely to experience the attacks endured by our previously referenced 7-year-old patient, Chris. Indeed, exposures to water damage, mold and mildew, pests like cockroaches and rodents, tobacco smoke, and pollutants are all known to make asthma worse [8–11]. As another example, we know that hunger and food insecurity are exceedingly common in this country. Roughly one in four children lives in food-insecure households, where a food-secure household is defined by the US Department of Agriculture (USDA) as "access by all people at all times to enough food for an active, healthy life" [12, 13]. The rate of food insecurity is likely to be even higher within at-risk, under-resourced populations served by many academic primary care centers [14, 15]. As such, identifying these types of triggers and risks, such as adverse housing and food insecurity, as part of routine screening is gaining favor as a key component of preventive, outpatient care and is also starting to be implemented in some inpatient settings [16–18].

Of course, identifying risks is one thing, but overcoming those risks is the ultimate goal. However, physicians and those working within clinical settings may not have the requisite expertise to act appropriately. Community partners, organizations, and agencies with needed, complementary expertise may be critical adjuvants to the services clinicians and medical professionals can provide.

An MLP is an interdisciplinary collaboration between a medical entity such as a clinic or hospital and a legal entity such as an attorney, legal aid office, or law school. MLP partners approach improving health for their target population by addressing risks related to the SDH. By helping medical partners to identify and address legal barriers that may cause or exacerbate health problems, legal professionals can be key members of the healthcare team [19, 20]. Since addressing these legal barriers, which are frequently synonymous with risks related to the SDH, often requires a multidisciplinary team approach, MLP is an important component of medical education in structural competence. Training medical students and residents in the MLP approach is an opportunity to impart to the next generation of physicians the knowledge, skills, and attitudes to recognize and address barriers to health on the patient, clinic/institution, and population levels [21, 22].

To illustrate this point, let us return to our case, this time, imagining that there was a legal advocate just down the hall for the resident to consult, and she offered to join the resident in their visit.

Section 3: Revisiting This Common Medical Case with Added Perspective

After you, the pediatric resident, left the room the last time, you realized you needed help. Yes, Chris' asthma symptoms were better, but you were really worried that he was at high risk of being rehospitalized in the future. Yes,

NOTICE TO ALL RESIDENTS

May 24, 2010

At this time all residents are not permitted to install any a/c units for your apartment.

Anyone with an a/c unit will be evicted immediately.

Thank you
Management

Fig. 1 Document posted on the door of your patients' apartment

Brianna's failing to thrive did not appear to have an organic cause, but you just could not understand why she was not growing. As you discussed these concerns with your preceptor, she suggested you go back to the room to obtain more history. She recommended posing questions to the family about their in-home exposures, their experience with their public benefits, and their ability to keep food on the table. She handed you a form with validated social history questions relevant to these and other SDH. She also showed you where, within the electronic health record, these same questions were referenced and could be documented [16, 17, 23, 24]. Armed with this guidance, you return to the patients' room.

Once again, you start with Chris. You ask him and his mother if they have thoughts about what might have triggered his asthma attack. Although Ms. Williams is unsure, she says Chris seems to be really sensitive to temperature swings. He has not been doing so well with the recent heat wave that has been hitting the city, especially considering that those occupying apartment units at her building have been told that they are not allowed to have window air conditioning units. She pulls out a paper she has in her purse, one that had been posted on her front door just days before (Fig. 1).

She also mentions that her apartment unit "is riddled with cockroaches, the ceiling is falling in, and [her] landlord isn't responsive to [her] concerns." She takes out her phone and shows you some pictures (Fig. 2).

You are horrified and do not know quite what to say. You thank her for her honesty and express your uncertainty at how to respond. You tell the mother that you would like to discuss this new information with your preceptor. First, however, you had a few more questions about Brianna. You ask Ms. Williams about whether she is currently receiving public benefits for herself, the family, or the infant. The mother notes that she has the Special Supplemental Nutrition Program for Women, Infants, and Children (WIC) [25] and has applied for SNAP (i.e., food stamps) [26], but she has not yet received her SNAP benefits and cannot determine the status of her application. You feel similarly confused, at a loss for how to continue. You excuse yourself from the room and return to your preceptor.

Fig. 2 Photograph of the home of your patients

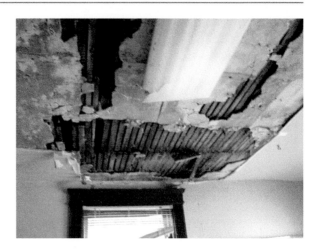

You tell your preceptor this new information, about how you think that, perhaps, the problems experienced by both Chris and Brianna may have their origins in these newly uncovered factors. Listening intently, your preceptor recommends that you speak with the legal advocate down the hall, who is a member of your clinic's MLP. This advocate has expertise in the legal rights of people with low income. You knock on their door curious about how they will add to your assessment and about whether they will be able to devise care plans that add value to your own. With the legal advocate, you review both of the cases and contemplate additional questions you might pose to the family, questions that may direct the legal care plan in more specific ways. You then go back to the room, explain to Ms. Williams that there are legal professionals right there in the clinic with expertise in some of the problems she is facing, and ask her if it would be okay to bring the advocate in to meet her. After she says yes, you return once again to the room, this time with the advocate by your side.

After introducing your partner from the MLP, the legal advocate jumps in with a clear awareness of some potentially important questions that build upon your assessment. She asks the mother, "What is your address? Who is the landlord? Has the local health or building department inspected your apartment for code violations?" Ms. Williams was initially surprised to learn she might get housing help at her children's doctor visit, but she is glad to speak with anyone who may be able to assist. She states that they live in a multiunit apartment building in a neighborhood just blocks from the hospital, one characterized by high rates of poverty and crime. No one has inspected their apartment for code violations. The legal advocate knows the area well and knows the landlord by reputation. You think to yourself that you would have never asked these questions, questions that already have led you down a far different path than where you were mere moments before.

With this new perspective, you are now curious about how the legal advocate will approach Brianna. She asks some quick follow-up questions relevant to the infant's case, focusing first on the family's benefits: "When did you apply? Have you turned in all the documentation on your household size and income that the public benefits office needs? What have they told you?" The mother replies that her application went in the same week Brianna was born and she has done everything the public benefits office asked. She has been bounced around from one caseworker to another whenever she has tried to follow up. As a result, the household is struggling to put food on the table. She is pleased that she has been able to continue breastfeeding Brianna, but she has been forced to feed Chris "Hamburger Helper" without the meat. As for herself, she is eating only oatmeal once or twice a day.

You step out of the room to let the legal advocate continue to obtain history from Ms. Williams and formulate her plan. You feel increasingly like albuterol alone will not help Chris and that a feeding diary for Brianna may be wholly insufficient. You relay what you just heard to your preceptor and the other residents and medical students in the office's workroom. You contemplate the breadth of what you just heard, the questions the advocate asked that you would not have considered. You had never thought of asking about the neighborhood, about the landlord, and about certain aspects of public benefits. You had never considered how to expand your social history to reach those social and environmental factors clearly at the core of your patients' experienced morbidity. How could that be changed? You find that even in the short time, you were with the legal advocate and you learned quite a bit. You make a mental note of key questions that you might pose to future patients to help you identify legal and structural barriers and consider making other MLP referrals.

Section 4: Co-developed Educational Curricula on the Social Determinants of Health

The questions that the resident started grappling with as described within the section above were posed at the primary care centers of Cincinnati Children's Hospital Medical Center (CCHMC) several years ago. What could and should families be screened for? Evidence suggests the majority of low-income families receiving care at urban pediatric clinics report at least one unmet basic need related to underlying poverty; many report several such needs [24, 27]. A recent survey at CCHMC highlighted that 28% of primary care families had their gas or electricity shut off in the previous year; 23% had doubled up (lived with others to pay the rent) or moved to a cheaper residence; 14% of mothers diluted their formula to make it last longer; and 33% had run out of food without money to buy more [14, 15].

Based on the information from these and other local surveys, risks related to the SDH have emerged as significant issues to be addressed consistently with families in the Pediatric Primary Care Center (PPCC) at CCHMC. The recognition of their importance grew alongside CCHMC's MLP, the Cincinnati Child Health-Law Partnership (Child HeLP), a partnership between the hospital's primary care centers and the nonprofit Legal Aid Society of Greater Cincinnati (Legal Aid) [28]. Child HeLP launched in 2008 to assist medical providers and social workers with helping patient-families resolve social and legal problems by adding legal advocates (i.e., attorneys and paralegals) from Legal Aid to the healthcare team [19]. SDH screening processes were initiated through the electronic health record and now routinely occur in over 90% of primary care encounters [16, 24]. Screening questions address housing conditions, food insecurity, public benefits denials and delays, mental health concerns, intimate partner violence, barriers to education, and availability of transportation. Questions were selected after a review of existing evidence and discussions with our key community partners, including legal advocates from the MLP. Questions were also tested for feedback from those that mattered most, patients and their families. The enhanced social screening processes enable clinicians and social workers to more effectively identify patients to refer to the MLP.

As the expanded social history was deployed and as Child HeLP developed and grew, curricula were put into place to train pediatric residents on the relevance and importance of the SDH. A series of didactic and experiential learning sessions were co-developed with medical and legal staff. The facilitated didactic sessions focus on legal rights (e.g., landlord-tenant laws, public benefits eligibility) and are delivered by an interdisciplinary team of pediatricians and legal advocates. Immersion experiences take learners out of the clinic and into the local public benefits office, a large food bank, and a neighborhood that is home to many PPCC patients. Within this neighborhood, learners meet local leaders (e.g., elementary school principal, community center manager) who paint a picture of what life is like within that community. To improve how SDH were discussed with patients, the team also has put into place a "video curriculum" that provides realistic examples of how to discuss social risks and resources with families. Videos include scenarios where interactions and interventions are solely medically based compared to those that also address underlying social issues. Videos include first-hand testimony from families as to how they experienced discussions of risks and ensuing actions (i.e., their experience with Child HeLP). Early evidence suggests that these educational pursuits have led to increased comfort by residents in addressing the SDH as well as more referrals to our available resources [16, 29–33]. These available resources, most notably Child HeLP, have led to key positive outcomes at both the patient and population levels [19, 34].

Section 5: Moving from Patient to Population Health Together

The legal advocate returns from her office to discuss next steps related to Chris and Brianna. After confirming that Ms. Williams has authorized her to discuss this information with you, she starts with Chris. She tells you that she immediately knew this complaint sounded familiar to her. A legal colleague had mentioned in passing just days earlier that one of her clients had reported that her landlord threatened eviction over putting in a window air conditioning unit. When the legal advocate went back to substantiate this in the Legal Aid case management database, to ensure that her memory served her well, she identified that this was not just a coincidence. It was an "outbreak" of substandard housing amenable to collective action. In the preceding weeks, there had been more than 15 referrals to Child HeLP from buildings managed by the same out-of-state landlord. Publically available city data suggested that each of the 19 complexes managed by this landlord had outstanding violations of city housing ordinances [34]. This "outbreak" called for action in the short and long terms. It also called for action for Chris and his family, as well as his neighbors and fellow tenants. In this sense, individual cases collectively highlighted a structural issue amenable to a structural intervention. This occurred because multiple cases were brought to the same partners, a key aspect of MLP enabling both individualized and population-wide action.

What about Chris' sister Brianna? What about the food insecurity that was also plaguing this family? The legal advocate had news there, too. After advocacy with the local public benefits office, she secured SNAP benefits for the family by the end of the day. Benefits were issued retroactively to the months since Ms. Williams's application was filed because of the county's failure to meet its legal duty to provide benefits in a timely manner. Ms. Williams received nearly $500.00 in food assistance that week and the confidence that she would be able to feed herself and her children moving forward.

Over time, Child HeLP's assistance continued for the Williams family had expanded to benefit other similarly situated families. For example, a Legal Aid attorney was connected to Ms. Williams and educated her on her legal rights to healthy housing and the process for filing an escrow case in court to legally withhold her rent payments until the landlord made legally required repairs. The attorney also filed complaints with the local health and building departments that enforce health and safety ordinances. This strategy was a clear example of "population justice" occurring in the confines of the primary care clinic. It was also a clear example of how patient health was quickly ratcheted up, becoming an indicator of population health; again a unique reality made possible by the MLP. Indeed, one child in one housing unit quickly expanded to include the other 15 units the MLP had identified, placing them within a larger cadre of nearly 700 low-income housing units that were at potential risk [34].

It is in this space that population health can be quickly linked to population justice (Fig. 3).

Collaborative work by the MLP led to this identification of a large cluster, an "outbreak," of substandard, poor-quality housing conditions. This collaborative response improved the housing situation for individual patients and families, and it also created linkages between tenants leading to meaningful community-wide housing improvements. Indeed, organization and advocacy promoted by the MLP led to improvements for both the "sick child" (Chris and other tenants with asthma who were patients of CCHMC) and the portfolio of more than 19 "sick buildings" (those managed by the out-of-state landlord). Here, asthma was a common health issue among the children identified by the MLP, but many other health problems are known to be associated with stress and with substandard housing in particular [10, 34].

Limiting or removing asthma triggers in housing units with high-risk children makes a difference. Over the months that followed, the MLP led building- and complex-wide activities devoted to improving home environmental conditions for

Population Health	**Population Justice**
Physician screens for food insecurity Clinic partners with foodbank to provide in-clinic supply of emergency infant formula	Legal advocate recovers delayed SNAP benefits MLP advocates for policy changes to get infants on benefits faster
Physician identifies housing concerns Clinic compiles health outcome data across high risk buildings	Legal advocate represents family to prevent eviction MLP facilitates formation of tenant association to pursue building-wide improvement
Physician identifies recent expulsion Clinic partners with local kindergarten readiness agencies	Legal advocate represents child at expulsion hearing MLP works with school district to reduce out-of-school discipline
Social worker talks with mother about intimate partner violence Clinic collaborates with agency around family support	Legal advocate helps get mother Civil Protection Order MLP participates in local alliance for women

Fig. 3 Linking population health with population justice to promote health and well-being

referred children and families as well as the broader tenant population. A team of Legal Aid attorneys and advocates helped to organize a tenant association and utilized litigation and other legal strategies to obtain substantial improvements. Of the 19 buildings in the out-of-state landlord's portfolio, 11 received significant systemic repairs (e.g., a new roof, new windows). This particular portfolio of buildings, which the absentee out-of-state landlord ultimately allowed to go into foreclosure, was subsequently purchased by a nonprofit developer. This new developer is now working with other community agencies, and a large grant from the Department of Housing and Urban Development, to rejuvenate these buildings inside and out. Legal Aid continued to advocate for further improvements and maintenance to ensure that the buildings are affordable and healthy.

Williams' situation also provided a means through which the MLP could facilitate a jump from patient to population and from population health to population justice in the area of nutrition and food security. The legal advocate and her colleagues saw this case, among others, as indicative of an alarming trend toward increasingly lengthy application processing delays for SNAP. Indeed, a large percentage of eligible families were not getting their applications for their public benefits approved by the 30-day deadline required by law. This observation was found to be part of a broader, system-wide issue, identified through Legal Aid's active surveillance of publically available data on the timeliness of public benefit application processing (i.e., time from application to decision). Then, through negotiation with the local public benefits agency, Legal Aid attorneys secured systemic changes in application processing procedures that resulted in a 30% increase in timely food assistance application decisions in just 4 months. Continued advocacy has greatly increased the numbers of applications processed in a timely fashion and ensured that other children and families in the community get the help they need to reduce food insecurity.

Section 6: A Common Medical (-Legal) Case with a Happy Outcome

It is a brisk fall morning. You are excited because today you will be following up with two of your favorite patients for their well-child checks – a now 8-year-old Chris and his now 7-month-old sister Brianna. Outside the room, you reflect on how your practice has changed in the past few months. Not only have you become more adept at screening for and addressing risks related to the SDH, but the ongoing broader advocacy undertaken by Child HeLP has also given you increased structural competency. You have come to understand and appreciate how existing systems – within the four walls of the primary care center and within the broader community – have a strong influence over the health of your patients. You have also watched as improvements to those various systems have directly resulted from advocacy by Child HeLP. It has been inspiring for you to be a part of that interdisciplinary team.

You enter the room and start with Chris, asking all the questions you have now grown accustomed to asking, considering those interventions, both medical and social, that are now part of your armamentarium. Chris has had a wonderful summer and a happy start to the school year. He says he wants to be a scientist. He has been taking his daily asthma controller medications without any issues and has rarely required his rescue medication. His home is free of cockroaches and the ceiling and walls of his home have been fixed. Ms. Williams states that repairs across the building are ongoing. Chris has not been to the emergency department since last spring.

You turn to Brianna who looks like a different baby. She continues to breastfeed and has also started to receive solid foods. She is back on the growth curve such that you would never know, just by looking at her, that she had ever failed to thrive. Ms. Williams appears healthier and happier, too. She tells you the family no longer goes without food – WIC and SNAP benefits are helping the family considerably. She and Chris are eating three meals a day; Ms. Williams only eats oatmeal when she wants to eat oatmeal. While you are talking, you smile as you hear Brianna babbling in the background. As you leave the room to place your orders, you walk by the Child HeLP office to express gratitude. You have come to understand that referrals to or consults of community experts are often just, if not more impactful, referrals to or consults of medical experts.

Conclusion

Clinical providers and legal advocates, as part of a broadly conceived healthcare team, can be an effective force for change. Indeed, attorneys and paralegals can help physicians and nurses understand social determinants. They can also partner with healthcare providers to use the law as a tool to address key risks, to intervene, and

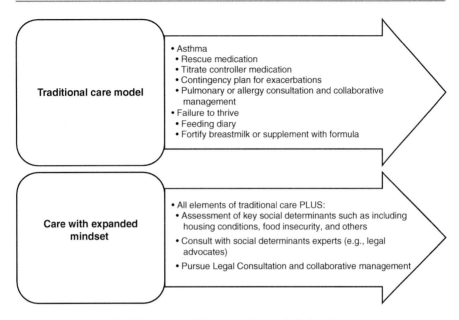

Fig. 4 Comparison of traditional care with a changed, more holistic mindset

to advocate for patients and families through interventions not yet typical in the clinical setting. Although medical trainees generally accept the importance of social and environmental exposures on health outcomes, many still focus narrowly on medical treatments despite the undeniable influence of contextual social and environmental factors (Fig. 4).

This case, and others like it [1], highlights how a broader mindset that considers both medical and social factors is critical to achieving desired outcomes and how bridging complementary areas of expertise (e.g., medicine and law) can support the health and well-being of patients and populations.

References

1. Tyler ET. In: Lawton E, Conroy K, Sandel M, Zuckerman B, editors. Poverty, health and law: readings and cases for medical-legal partnership. 1st ed. Durham: Carolina Academic Press; 2011.
2. Williams DR, Sternthal M, Wright RJ. Social determinants: taking the social context of asthma seriously. Pediatrics. 2009;123(Suppl 3):S174–84.
3. Suglia SF, Franco Suglia S, Duarte CS, Sandel MT, Wright RJ. Social and environmental stressors in the home and childhood asthma. J Epidemiol Community Health. 2010;64(7):636–42.
4. Sandel M, Wright RJ. When home is where the stress is: expanding the dimensions of housing that influence asthma morbidity. Arch Dis Child. 2006;91(11):942–8.
5. Beck AF, Huang B, Chundur R, Kahn RS. Housing code violation density associated with emergency department and hospital use by children with asthma. Health Aff (Millwood). 2014;33(11):1993–2002.

6. Akinbami LJ, Moorman JE, Simon AE, Schoendorf KC. Trends in racial disparities for asthma outcomes among children 0 to 17 years, 2001–2010. J Allergy Clin Immunol. 2014;134(3):547–53.e5.
7. Moorman JE, Akinbami LJ, Bailey CM, Zahran HS, King ME, Johnson CA, et al. National surveillance of asthma: United States, 2001–2010. Vital Health Stat. 3. 2012;35:1–58.
8. Crocker DD, Kinyota S, Dumitru GG, Ligon CB, Herman EJ, Ferdinands JM, et al. Effectiveness of home-based, multi-trigger, multicomponent interventions with an environmental focus for reducing asthma morbidity: a community guide systematic review. Am J Prev Med. 2011;41(2. Suppl 1):S5–32.
9. Rosenfeld L, Rudd R, Chew GL, Emmons K, Acevedo-García D. Are neighborhood-level characteristics associated with indoor allergens in the household? J Asthma. 2010;47(1):66–75.
10. Saegert SC, Klitzman S, Freudenberg N, Cooperman-Mroczek J, Nassar S. Healthy housing: a structured review of published evaluations of US interventions to improve health by modifying housing in the United States, 1990–2001. Am J Public Health. 2003;93(9):1471–7.
11. Newman NC, Ryan PH, Huang B, Beck AF, Sauers HS, Kahn RS. Traffic-related air pollution and asthma hospital readmission in children: a longitudinal cohort study. J Pediatr. 2014;164(6):1396–402.e1.
12. Coleman-Jensen A, Gregory CA, Singh A. Household food security in the United States in 2013 [Internet]. [cited 2018 Oct 3]. Available from: https://www.ers.usda.gov/publications/pub-details/?pubid=45268
13. Map the Meal Gap [Internet]. Feeding America. [cited 2018 Oct 3]. Available from: http://map.feedingamerica.org//
14. Burkhardt MC, Beck AF, Kahn RS, Klein MD. Are our babies hungry? food insecurity among infants in urban clinics. Clin Pediatr (Phila). 2012;51(3):238–43.
15. DeMartini TL, Beck AF, Kahn RS, Klein MD. Food insecure families: description of access and barriers to food from one pediatric primary care center. J Community Health. 2013;38(6):1182–7.
16. Burkhardt MC, Beck AF, Conway PH, Kahn RS, Klein MD. Enhancing accurate identification of food insecurity using quality-improvement techniques. Pediatrics. 2012;129(2):e504–10.
17. Beck AF, Sauers HS, Kahn RS, Yau C, Weiser J, Simmons JM. Improved documentation and care planning with an asthma-specific history and physical. Hosp Pediatr. 2012;2(4):194–201.
18. Colvin JD, Bettenhausen JL, Anderson-Carpenter KD, Collie-Akers V, Plencner L, Krager M, et al. Multiple behavior change intervention to improve detection of unmet social needs and resulting resource referrals. Acad Pediatr. 2016;16(2):168–74.
19. Klein MD, Beck AF, Henize AW, Parrish DS, Fink EE, Kahn RS. Doctors and lawyers collaborating to HeLP children – outcomes from a successful partnership between professions. J Health Care Poor Underserved. 2013;24(3):1063–73.
20. Sandel M, Hansen M, Kahn R, et al. Medical-legal partnerships: transforming primary care by addressing the legal needs of vulnerable populations. Health Aff (Millwood). 2010;29(9):1697–705.
21. Paul EG, Curran M, Tobin Tyler E. The medical-legal partnership approach to teaching social determinants of health and structural competency in residency programs. Acad Med. 2017;92(3):292–8.
22. Tobin-Tyler E, Teitelbaum J. Training the 21st-century health care team: maximizing interprofessional education through medical-legal partnership. Acad Med. 2016;91(6):761–5.
23. Chung EK, Siegel BS, Garg A, et al. Screening for social determinants of health among children and families living in poverty: a guide for clinicians. Curr Probl Pediatr Adolesc Health Care. 2016;46(5):135–53.
24. Beck AF, Klein MD, Kahn RS. Identifying social risk via a clinical social history embedded in the electronic health record. Clin Pediatr (Phila). 2012;51(10):972–7.
25. Women, Infants, and Children (WIC) ǀ Food and Nutrition Service [Internet]. [cited 2018 Oct 3]. Available from: https://www.fns.usda.gov/wic/women-infants-and-children-wic

26. Garg A, Butz AM, Dworkin PH, Lewis RA, Thompson RE, Serwint JR. Improving the management of family psychosocial problems at low-income children's well-child care visits: the WE CARE Project. Pediatrics. 2007;120(3):547–58.
27. Child HeLP (Legal Aid) | General and Community Pediatrics [Internet]. [cited 2018 Oct 3]. Available from: https://www.cincinnatichildrens.org/service/g/gen-pediatrics/services/child-help
28. Real FJ, Michelson CD, Beck AF, Klein MD. Location, location, location: teaching about neighborhoods in pediatrics. Acad Pediatr. 2017;17(3):228–32.
29. Real FJ, Beck AF, Spaulding JR, Sucharew H, Klein MD. Impact of a neighborhood-based curriculum on the helpfulness of pediatric Residents' anticipatory guidance to impoverished families. Matern Child Health J. 2016;20(11):2261–7.
30. Klein MD, Alcamo AM, Beck AF, et al. Can a video curriculum on the social determinants of health affect residents' practice and families' perceptions of care? Acad Pediatr. 2014;14(2):159–66.
31. O'Toole JK, Burkhardt MC, Solan LG, Vaughn L, Klein MD. Resident confidence addressing social history: is it influenced by availability of social and legal resources? Clin Pediatr (Phila). 2012;51(7):625–31.
32. O'Toole JK, Solan LG, Burkhardt MC, Klein MD. Watch and learn: an innovative video trigger curriculum to increase resident screening for social determinants of health. Clin Pediatr (Phila). 2013;52(4):344–50.
33. Beck AF, Henize AW, Kahn RS, Reiber KL, Young JJ, Klein MD. Forging a pediatric primary care-community partnership to support food-insecure families. Pediatrics. 2014;134(2):e564–71.
34. Beck AF, Klein MD, Schaffzin JK, Tallent V, Gillam M, Kahn RS. Identifying and treating a substandard housing cluster using a medical-legal partnership. Pediatrics. 2012;130(5):831–8.

Part III

Structural Competency in Community Engagement

Program for Residency Education, Community Engagement, and Peer Support Training (PRECEPT): Connecting Psychiatrists to Community Resources in Harlem, NYC

Selena Suhail-Sindhu, Parth Patel, Judith Sugarman, and Helena Hansen

The Problem

Stark inequalities in the diagnosis, treatment, and outcome of disabling serious mental illnesses (SMI) by race, ethnicity, and socioeconomic status are well established [1–3]. These conditions are associated with frequent use of emergency and inpatient care and with a heavy burden of morbidity and mortality in low-income communities of color [4]. The social conditions of those living with SMI, such as unstable housing and income, low availability of supportive social networks, heightened stigma, and exclusion, are rooted at the intersection of race and social class and are predictive of poor mental health outcomes [5–7]. Conversely, the positive relationship of social services (e.g., housing and employment) and community support (e.g., in clubhouses, faith-based and cultural organizations, as well as peer navigation) to mental health outcomes is well established [8–11].

Yet, clinics and practitioners are often disconnected from community resources and receive little training and guidance on strategies to identify and address social determinants of health that have a direct relationship to poor mental health outcomes. These daunting work conditions contribute to professional burnout and shortages of psychiatrists in the public mental health system [12–14]. The combination of public workforce shortages, the stigma of mental illness, poor clinician understandings of

S. Suhail-Sindhu · H. Hansen (✉)
New York University, New York City, NY, USA
e-mail: helena.hansen@nyumc.org

P. Patel
Mount Sinai Medical Center, Miami Beach, FL, USA

J. Sugarman
Center for Urban and Community Services, New York, NY, USA

© Springer Nature Switzerland AG 2019
H. Hansen, J. M. Metzl (eds.), *Structural Competency in Mental Health and Medicine*,
https://doi.org/10.1007/978-3-030-10525-9_11

the social context of mental health inequities, and gaps between clinical and social service systems leads to persistent cycles of health disparities and trauma for those with SMI. These challenges underscore the value of aligning mental healthcare services with community and social resources for patients with SMI, which also enables, engages, and helps to retain clinicians in public psychiatry. Stated another way, structures (and their fragmentation) that overdetermine poor health outcomes, and thus foster the cynicism of practitioners, call on practitioners to participate in altering the structures themselves. Here we describe an initiative that does this by training psychiatrists to bridge clinical care with community resources.

Theoretical Framework

Physician leadership and multidisciplinary collaboration are needed to address the institutional roots of health disparities and develop trust with community members [15]. Increasingly, psychiatrists do not work as solo practitioners, but rather serve as medical directors of multidisciplinary teams, responsible for coordinating diverse team members including those specialized in community and social services. Psychiatrists and their clinical teams are therefore charged with diagnosing and treating the social, as well as biological, bases of their patients' distress. This calls for *structural competency*, for intervention above the level of individual patients, through partnerships with community agencies and non-health sectors—such as schools, policing, and housing—to develop resource networks that promote health [16–18].

This requires a paradigm shift, because mental health practitioners are currently trained to interpret individual-level causation. The *explanatory model* [19] of psychiatrists attributes mental health problems to physiological/genetic substrates and individual behavioral conditioning. Mental health practitioners (including clinical social workers and case managers) working in this individualist frame narrowly focus on medication management, behavioral counseling, and appointment adherence. Their training does not allow them to integrate community-based resources and peer support into patient care. To incorporate social determinants of health in their explanatory model and problem-solving approach, psychiatrists, therapists, counselors, and social workers must be taught to see patient's health problems in terms of their structural/environmental causes—within a *social ecological model* [20]—and to partner with other disciplines and community organizations with resources to intervene on social conditions. Since clinicians learn primarily through modeling and practice rather than in classrooms, such a shift in explanatory model and intervention will require meaningful contact with community agencies, as well as guidance to identify and use community resources.

Peers as Facilitators of Engagement with Community Agencies

Trained peers—also referred to as those with lived experience of psychiatric diagnosis—who have successfully navigated complex social and health service systems have unique experiential knowledge and skills, as well as a shared lived context of the intersection of disease and social exclusions. Peer mental health workers and navigators serve as trusted bridges and sources of information for patients living with illness and powerful role models for recovery. Studies have demonstrated peers' effectiveness in early engagement and in promoting patients' community support and treatment adherence [21–23].

New York State (NYS) serves as a laboratory for peer mental health workers in public clinics. NYS' Medicaid redesign program includes reimbursement categories and new licensing procedures for peer mental health workers. New York City (NYC) hosted the country's first major clinical trial of a community-based alternative to hospitalization for people in psychiatric crisis, featuring peer workers in community respite centers [24]. The trial documented the crucial role of peers in care coordination and also the need to train psychiatrists in delivery of multidisciplinary care which includes peers, given psychiatrists' legal liability for clinical decisions, and psychiatrists' uncertainty about the role of peers and how to effectively integrate peers into clinical care teams. In community-based mental health clinics, peer mental health workers who have personal experience and success with navigating community resources are untapped potential facilitators for connecting clinical teams with community partners, but they are seldom part of mental health treatment planning, and mental health practitioners need explicit training in how to collaborate with peers.

The Path: Community Engagement and Peer Collaboration

The PRECEPT project is a dynamic, evolving program which is required for all second year (PGY2) psychiatry residents at New York University (NYU) that incorporates ethnographic fieldwork, community engagement and resource mapping, structural competency training, and the opportunity to collaborate with a peer mental health specialist. In a collaboration between the NYU psychiatry residency training program and the Manhattan Psychiatric Center (MPC), PRECEPT is based out of the MPC outpatient mental health clinic on 125th street and Adam Clayton Powell Boulevard in which psychiatry residents treat patients; however PRECEPT brings psychiatrists outside of the clinic through site visits to organizations throughout Harlem and surrounding neighborhoods. NYU second year psychiatry residents engage in a 6-week rotation at the 125th street clinic where elements of PRECEPT are weaved throughout their weekly clinical work. Come Friday afternoon, the residents leave the clinic space for a different learning environment in the surrounding neighborhoods that is, as we will describe, equally as critical as any that make up the majority of their clinical studies and training.

For the first 2 years, the core of our PRECEPT team was comprised of a peer specialist with lived experience of a psychiatric diagnosis who also had ethnographic mental health research training, a graduate level public health researcher, and an undergraduate pre-medicine anthropology student with skills in mapping software and design. The faculty supervisor for PRECEPT was a psychiatrist-anthropologist uniquely positioned to lead introductory discussions of the concepts of structural competency and peer support and to advocate for PRECEPT to be required for all second year residents in the training program and clinical curriculum. The breadth of skills, educational backgrounds, and experiences represented in our team is the kind of creative collaboration often necessary for meaningful work in structural competency training and effective structural interventions. Inherent to our group is the idea that psychiatry residents, public health researchers, anthropology students, and peers can learn from and teach one another in order to address the larger structural issues that affect the course of mental illness and recovery, particularly in communities where resources can be scarce and socioeconomic and political inequalities can have very real health effects. Below, we describe the different components of PRECEPT as well as two significant phases of the project that have evolved out of the day-to-day iterative process of trying to radically reimagine what the scope of a clinician's role might be.

Practicing Psychiatry in Harlem: A Lesson in History, Built Environment, and Racial Inequality

The 125th street clinic bases our project in Harlem, a historically African-American neighborhood with a history of racial inequalities and deprivation through policies such as redlining that can still be felt today. The clinic is located at a crossroads between East Harlem, also known as Spanish Harlem, with a large number of Latino residents, and West Harlem, with largely African-American residents—neighborhoods with different demographics, resources, and mixed income levels. These differences become mapped onto the physical environment of Harlem in conspicuous ways, and because much of the work and learning done through PRECEPT takes place on foot, residents have a chance to reflect upon the changing scenery. Walking east on 125th street from the clinic, newer buildings and businesses targeted toward more affluent newcomers gradually give way to boarded up storefronts, fast-food chains, and the ominous remnants of a long-closed grocery store. Our team allows for space to discuss the varying built environment of Harlem that the psychiatry residents might observe, in relation to the cultural and political economic history of Harlem. We come back to these conversations as a team when later in the 6-week rotation, we drop by a harm reduction center on the east side of town. Newly attuned to structural issues, residents can now connect their observation that services such as harm reduction centers and methadone clinics seem more concentrated in East Harlem with the fact that this area also has higher rates of poverty, unemployment, and a history of underinvestment from the city including long-standing racially discriminatory lending practices preventing home and business ownership by African-American and Latino residents (Fig. 1). Patients seen at the clinic that may have a dual diagnosis with substance abuse and are referred to these services are now placed in a broader structural reality rather than seen solely as individuals struggling with addiction.

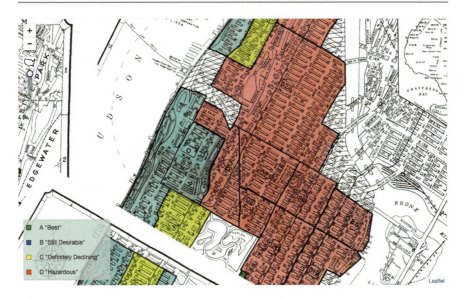

Fig. 1 A map of redlining in Harlem and Upper Manhattan (Home Owners' Loan Corporation residential security map, 1938). Redlining was a practice of banks and lending institutions of designating "high-risk" (in red) zones ineligible for mortgage or small business loans, and "risk" was largely gauged by the percentage of residents that were ethnic and racial minorities and recent immigrants. In PRECEPT, psychiatry residents are asked to locate the clinic and assess whether areas labeled in red as "high risk" are still less prosperous today based on their fieldwork

PRECEPT has also taken place during a period of rapid gentrification in Harlem that has changed our project over time. For example, early on in the initial rotations, we asked residents to take a walk throughout the neighborhood and return to the clinic with fresh grapes. Residents came back empty-handed after experiencing a little bit of what it means to live in a "food desert"—that is, until a new Whole Foods opened one block from the clinic after the first year of PRECEPT, representing changes in the food environment associated with gentrification.

Given that the psychiatry residents primarily work at and around NYU Langone Medical Center and Bellevue Hospital in the Midtown East area of Manhattan, many had not ventured uptown into Harlem before. For the majority of the residents, this 6-week rotation was the first time they had spent any significant amount of time in Harlem. With wide differences in race, socioeconomic status, and education levels of the residents compared to their patients seen at the 125th clinic, most of whom are African American or Latino and Medicaid recipients and diagnosed as "severely mentally ill," the introductory week of PRECEPT is dedicated to a community walk and a visit to an arts and cultural center in Harlem. The Black Power exhibit at the Schomburg Center for Research on Black Culture on 135th street provides a history of civil rights movements in the USA and NYC. Residents are often surprised to learn how central health activism was to the Black Panther Party and the Young Lords, groups that worked to secure greater healthcare access and resources for their communities. Contemporary art exhibits at the Studio Museum in Harlem comment on timely issues of racism and inequality, mass incarceration, and capitalism that opened up space for residents to discuss issues of race, privilege, and power that can often be difficult for clinicians to engage with, as well as conversations about what it means from a structural and individual level to live and practice medicine in a for-profit healthcare system.

Phase I: Exploratory Fieldwork, Qualitative Research, and Peer Collaboration

A main component of PRECEPT is community fieldwork in Harlem that entails site visits to community-based organizations, outpatient clinics, and social service organizations that provide mental and physical healthcare treatment and access or have some role in the well-being of the community. Fieldwork was initially "exploratory," meaning visits to various organizations and sites were not necessarily scheduled beforehand and a great emphasis was placed on building relationships as a team with organizations in the community over time. This approach was inspired by the anthropological research method of ethnography, where individuals spend time in a community to build relationships and understand local forms of knowledge and culture. Sites visited in Harlem included mental health outpatient clinics, homeless shelters, harm reduction centers, soup kitchens and food banks, transitional living residences, and community rights groups. Other sites that expanded residents' definition of "community engagement" included places such as community gardens, senior citizen centers, churches, hair salons and other local small business, and clubhouses. We also explored residents' interests by providing examples of structural level work in relation to their future clinical specialties in psychiatry. For example, we visited a criminal justice rights organization with a resident who was interested in pursuing forensic psychiatry, who learned about the role a psychiatrist could play at the intersection of mental healthcare and the justice system. Another resident who was interested in public policy relevant to mental healthcare met with a group of public psychiatrists actively engaged in integrating supportive housing into psychiatric care.

Psychiatry residents assisted us with qualitative interviews of community psychiatrists, social workers, peer mental health specialists, and a variety of other key informants working in organizations throughout Harlem. Together with residents, we developed a semi-structured interview guide. Topics included perceptions of mental health and recovery in the community, the everyday work of peer mental health specialists, and the facilitators and barriers to providing and accessing psychiatric services in Harlem and NYC.

Fundamental to PRECEPT has also been a "flipped" learning environment in which residents learn formally and informally from a peer mental health specialist on our team. Peers are individuals with lived experience with mental illness that work to engage other patients in their own recovery and work on clinical teams to tailor patient care. The majority of psychiatry residents had not worked closely with a peer. The peer who helped to develop PRECEPT engaged residents with humor and her own lived experience and opened up space for discussion of potentially controversial and sensitive issues in psychiatry such as patient rights, involuntary treatment, and the downsides of psychotropic medications. Having a peer teach psychiatrists-in-training has been an intentional effort to flip traditional hierarchies in medicine in which individuals with greater clinical education have the most authority. Below is an excerpt from our first peer instructor's personal narrative, which she routinely shared with psychiatry residents when first meeting them, first as a written, anonymous document, and then disclosing after having residents read and respond to it that it described her own life:

> *Five generations of my family have been diagnosed with serious mental illness. When I was a kid, alongside the vitamins on our kitchen table I saw pills with the names stelazine, thorazine, etrafon and trilafon, and a rainbow of other medications. By the age of 13 I was addicted to narcotics. My parents pharmaceutically withdrew, so I attached myself to my classical bass teacher, was admitted to a world renown music school, but dropped out because of a paralyzing depression. A decade later, I lost custody of my son after multiple hospitalizations. I was put in four point restraints and had ECT. Then, at 45 years old, I was finally, accurately diagnosed with bipolar II.*
>
> *In one fell swoop, I went from having depression—the common cold of mental illness – to serious mental illness: bipolar. I shared that diagnosis with mass murderers, folks with special relationships with God, people who ran naked in the street.*
>
> *I would have given ANYTHING to meet someone who had experienced what I was going through—someone who was now comfortable in his or her own skin and living a decent and dignified life. Someone who could answer questions such as: How do I distinguish between my personality, my temperament, and my illness? Will I ever date again? Should I disclose my diagnosis on a date or at work? Will I be able to trust myself again when I have lost everything because of my psychotic episode?*
>
> *No one should have to face these questions alone.*
>
> *The first time I was hospitalized, the doctor who did my intake interview told me that if I wanted to get well I would have to change professions. I should find a job with more consistent hours. What she didn't know, **because she never asked**, was that before I entered the hospital, all that kept me from jumping out of my 22nd floor apartment was reading my own resume. On that piece of paper, I had a record of reality. I had been in 12 orchestras, and I told myself that no one would hire me if I were not competent. This hospital-doctor, who had met me half an hour prior, was telling me to ditch 32 years of my professional life and the largest component of my identity!*

Conversations about the role of peers in mental healthcare often extend over lunch, shared by the PRECEPT instructors including the peer and participating residents prior to fieldwork visits. At least once in every rotation, we are joined by a guest speaker who is often a peer at a community-based organization or clinic. At times, these conversations are difficult for residents who may feel personally criticized when hearing peers' stories of forced medication, verbal abuse, or stigmatization by professionals in the mental health system. In those cases, it has helped residents to debrief with other PRECEPT instructors. Informal teaching moments such as lunch conversations and during fieldwork in surrounding neighborhoods have been crucial to helping psychiatry residents integrate knowledge of structural issues that they may otherwise find overwhelming or outside the scope of their work as psychiatrists.

Phase II: Structured Didactics and Planned Site Visits

After receiving feedback from residents that the uncertain nature of spontaneous community site visits was challenging, given the residents' desire for predictability and their habituation to office visits rather than exploratory field work, we adjusted our approach by pre-scheduling structured site visits. Residents preferred to be expected for a visit at a particular organization or agency over our previous approach of community engagement through neighborhood walks and unplanned site visits in an effort to identify new resources in Harlem. We reduced the variety of sites that we visited within a 6-week rotation, as we relied on organizations with which we had prior relationships to provide tours and informational sessions. However, this also increased the residents' comfort and engagement with scheduled visits.

In this second phase, we've also introduced more structure into our program by developing formal didactics on topics relevant to PRECEPT. Didactic topics include the history of Harlem, the deinstitutionalization in mental healthcare, the history of the mental health recovery movement, and the incorporation of peers in mental healthcare, distributed over the 6-week rotation. Residents have responded well to lectures on topics they may have only tangentially discussed in other areas of training and are able to connect these lessons to our fieldwork and community engagement.

Peer collaboration has continued through the second phase of PRECEPT. Residents have expressed enthusiasm about the opportunity to build a relationship with a peer mental health specialist in an informal setting in which peers teach residents about community-based care based on their personal and professional experiences.

Structural Intervention: Community Resource Map

Often in structural competency initiatives, students and clinical trainees become overwhelmed at the weight of a greater understanding of structural issues and feel helpless in addressing them through existing clinical knowledge and training. Trainees learn to connect social, political, and economic domains to clinical outcomes and, therefore, to clinical care, but these broad domains can seem overwhelming.

In order to produce a tangible, practical intervention from community engagement efforts and structural didactics, PRECEPT and participating residents developed a community resource map (Fig. 2) from the data collected during site visits, for use by clinical teams in treatment planning and social service referrals and ultimately to be used directly by patients. The community resource map is regularly updated by the PRECEPT team and residents based on fieldwork in Harlem and surrounding neighborhoods. Resources recorded in the resource map reflect organizations with which the team has built personal relationships. They are familiar with the 125th street clinic and its patients' needs and are invested in building a stronger network of services and organizations in Harlem. Many of these organizations have expressed interest in referring people in need of mental healthcare back to the 125th street clinic and coordinating services with the clinical staff; facilitating this coordination is a planned future focus of PRECEPT.

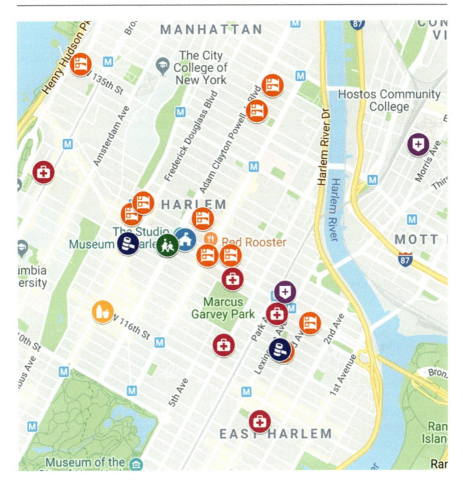

Fig. 2 Screenshot of interactive community resource map of Harlem. Icons indicate different types of services and organizations, such as homeless shelters, legal aid organizations, or outpatient primary care clinics. Clicking on each icon reveals a brief description of services, referral, and contact information for each organization

Psychiatry residents have been enthusiastic about creating and utilizing the map at the clinic, stating that previously, clinicians would refer patients who live in Harlem to far away areas because they were unaware of services in Harlem. Our fieldwork has allowed us to do the on-the-ground work to engage with community resources that clinicians, social workers, and other health professionals are unable to do from inside clinic walls. Giving psychiatry residents the opportunity to engage in a practical community engagement initiative has been critical in expanding structural competency into a set of practical tools, including skills in conducting fieldwork, building community relations, and creating more holistic treatment plans that incorporate community resources, in addition to theoretical knowledge.

Key Learnings

The different iterations of PRECEPT have caused us to think more critically about how to engage psychiatry residents in structural competency work, particularly of the kind that takes residents outside of the familiarity of clinical spaces and into potentially unfamiliar community spaces. Throughout PRECEPT, uncertainty was an inherent aspect of fieldwork and community engagement. The unstructured nature of exploring resources in Harlem led to genuine connections with individuals and organizations in the community. For example, our fieldwork showed us that individuals running community organizations who had not had prior contact with mental health practitioners were often excited to see clinicians taking an interest in their work. On the other hand, pre-scheduled site visits gave organizations an opportunity to give residents formal tours. In one instance, a harm reduction center was able to provide opioid overdose prevention kit (naloxone) training and certification to residents as a part of their tour. In the end, we opted for a compromise in which many site visits were scheduled in advance in order to increase residents' comfort with venturing into surrounding neighborhoods.

Some residents felt uncomfortable hearing about negative experiences of peers that implied criticisms of psychiatry, the role of medications, or the lack of care showed to patients by members of clinical teams. We learned that these conversations should be approached with sensitivity and may be best facilitated by experienced community psychiatrists who can help residents to put these reports in perspective as advice on how to be respectful of patients rather than as personal criticisms. Similarly, public psychiatrists are uniquely poised to help residents see the connection between structural level interventions into clinically relevant outcomes. Such connections are critical in helping clinical trainees to adopting structural competency frameworks in their thinking and practice.

Finally, doing fieldwork and engagement in low-income communities can be challenging for trainees who come from affluent backgrounds. Some psychiatry residents were hesitant to explore poor, predominately nonwhite neighborhoods such as East Harlem. While residents may be comfortable seeing patients from such communities in the controlled environments of clinics and hospitals where there are clear power hierarchies, they may be uncomfortable in the unknown territory of patients' neighborhoods. The accompaniment and guidance of PRECEPT team members, including peers, helped residents to overcome their fear, and most residents ultimately appreciated seeing where community-based organizations were located, what they looked like, and how they functioned and appreciated meeting their staff in order to inform their referrals from hospitals or clinics. Many residents stated that they would have wanted to be introduced to concepts from PRECEPT earlier in their clinical training. In fact a curriculum development advisory group of residents recommended to the residency director that PRECEPT should be introduced during their first year of residency, a year in which residents spend most of their time on emergency and inpatient units, where they do not get a sense of the community contexts from which their patients come, and are discouraged by the disconnectedness of their patients and the apparent futility of their clinical care.

This feedback from residents suggests that community engagement and collaboration with peers can indeed foster an enthusiasm for public psychiatry and optimism about the potential for structural interventions to improve mental health outcomes.

References

1. Office of the Surgeon General (US); Center for Mental Health Services (US); National Institute of Mental Health (US). Mental health: culture, race, and ethnicity: a supplement to mental health: a report of the surgeon general. Rockville: Substance Abuse and Mental Health Services Administration (US); 2001.
2. McGuire TG, Miranda J. Racial and ethnic disparities in mental health care: evidence and policy implications. Health Aff (Project Hope). 2008;27(2):393–403. https://doi.org/10.1377/hlthaff.27.2.393.
3. Safran M, Mays R, Huang L, McCuan R, Pham P, Fisher S, McDuffie K, Trachtenberg A. Mental health disparities. Am J Public Health. 2009;99(11):1962–6.
4. Walker ER, McGee RE, Druss BG. Mortality in mental disorders and global disease burden implications: a systematic review and meta-analysis. JAMA Psychiat. 2015;72(4):334–41.
5. Benston EA. Housing programs for homeless individuals with mental illness: effects on housing and mental health outcomes. Psychiatr Serv. 2015;66(8):806–16.
6. Palumbo C, Volpe U, Matanov A, Priebe S, Giacco D. Social networks of patients with psychosis: a systematic review. BMC Res Notes. 2015;8:560.
7. Schnyder N, Panczak R, Groth N, Schultze-Lutter F. Association between mental health-related stigma and active help-seeking: systematic review and meta-analysis. Br J Psychiatry. 2017;210(4):261–8.
8. Aubry T, Nelson G, Tsemberis S. Housing first for people with severe mental illness who are homeless: a review of the research and findings from the at home-chez soi demonstration project. Can J Psychiatr. 2015;60(11):467–74.
9. Latimer EA. Economic impacts of supported employment for persons with severe mental illness. Can J Psychiatr. 2001;46(6):496–505.
10. Anderson K, Laxhman N, Priebe S. Can mental health interventions change social networks? A systematic review. BMC Psychiatry. 2015;15:297.
11. Galanter M. The concept of spirituality in relation to addiction recovery and general psychiatry. Recent Dev Alcohol. 2008;18:125–40.
12. New York State Department of Health. Program overview and background: doctors across New York, physician practice support and physician loan repayment programs cycle IV. 2016. https://www.health.ny.gov/professionals/doctors/graduate_medical_education/doctors_across_ny/background.htm
13. Krupka C. Nearly half of physicians struggle with burnout. AMA News. September 3, 2012. http://www.amednews.com/article/20120903/profession/309039952/2/
14. Dyrbye LN, Tait SD. Physician burnout: a potential threat to successful health care reform. JAMA. 2011;305(19):2009–10.
15. Clancy G. Understanding deficiencies in leadership in advancing health equity: a case of pit bulls, public health, and pimps. Acad Med. 2015;90:418–20.
16. Metzl JM, Hansen H. Structural competency: theorizing a new medical engagement with stigma and inequality. Soc Sci Med. 2014;103:126–33.
17. Hansen H, Rohrbaugh R, Braslow J. Structural competency for psychiatry residents: a call to act on systemic discrimination and institutional racism. JAMA Psychiat. 2018;75(2):117–8.
18. Hansen H, Metzl J. New medicine for US health reform: training physicians for structural interventions. Acad Med. 2017;92(3):279–81.
19. Kleinman A, Benson P. Anthropology in the clinic: the problem of cultural competency and how to fix it. PLoS Med. 2006;3(10):e294.

20. CDC. Social ecological model: a framework for prevention. March 25, 2015. http://www.cdc. gov/ViolencePrevention/overview/social-ecologicalmodel.html
21. Davidson L, Bellamy C, Guy K, Miller R. Peer support among persons with severe mental illnesses: a review of evidence and experience. World Psychiatry. 2012;11:2.
22. Repper C, Carter R. A review of the literature on peer support in mental health services. J Ment Health. 2011;20(4):392–411.
23. Chinman M, George P, Dougherty R, Daniels A, Ghose S, Swift A, Delphin-Rittmon M. Peer support services for individuals with serious mental illnesses: assessing the evidence. Psychiatr Serv. 2014;65(4):429–41.
24. New York City Department of Health. Parachute NYC: tracing the origins, development, and implementation of an innovative alternative to psychiatric crisis. White Paper December 18, 2015.

Relational Politics of Clinical Care: Lessons from the University of California PRIME-LC Program

Michael J. Montoya

The Question

Wouldn't it be amazing if your physician had the time to listen to you? Not the kind of listening where they are trying to get your words to fit into a formula for the chart or a presentation. But a deep listening to *your* insight and experience, the conditions of your life, and the ways these tie in to the reason you came to see them. Even though the time constraints of a doctor's visit seem to prevent such an encounter, deep listening takes no more time than any other kind of listening. It is a quality of listening. The question then becomes, how can you teach medical students to deeply listen, to augment their training, within constraints of time, when considering clinical care options? This is what we are asking when we invite or require students to consider structure and equity in their clinical encounters. Deep listening occurs when a person tells their story, and we receive it attentively as a form of expertise about their injury, illness, and resources. Such listening elicits clues to a person's experiences and social environment, which are aspects of structural awareness. For students and early career physicians, the educational pressures, much more so clinical pressures to follow protocols, almost guarantee a posture of rigidity. And this posture it seems can only be shed, and very carefully so, after years of clinical practice. This essay offers a relational approach that uses humility as a key to unlocking postures toward patients that in turn enable deep listening and structural awareness. The approach has been developed through my work with first, second, and third year medical students and residents. I was hired in 2004 as the founding faculty for the Program in Medical Education for the Latino Community (PRIME-LC), a

M. J. Montoya (✉)
Anthropology & Chicanx/Latinx Studies, School of Social Sciences, Program in Medical Education for the Latino Community, School of Medicine, Public Health & Nursing Science, College of Health Sciences, University of California, Irvine, Irvine, CA, USA
e-mail: mmontoya@uci.edu

state-funded expansion of the medical school cohort for students committed to working with the Spanish-speaking medically underserved. I was recruited to PRIME-LC because my work examines the ways bioclinical science systematically cleaves the social from the biological for conditions like type 2 diabetes with obvious and well-accepted ecological preconditions [1].

Deep Listening

"I'm sorry Professor Montoya," the third year medical student (MSIII) in my seminar said, "But if you don't have an MD, no one is going to listen to you." We had been reading Jonathan M. Metzl and Helena Hansen's piece on structural competency [2], and students were acknowledging their frustration with the gulf between our course insights and their experiences on the wards. The course uses a variety of readings from the medical social sciences to introduce medical students to the social forces that affect health and health care, especially for Spanish-speaking patients. The course also is designed, through guided facilitated reflection, to prepare future physicians to be advocates for better clinical care and health equity in their practices. No one but me seemed to notice the paradox the student had brought to the discussion. I had, after all, assigned each reading for the express purpose of helping students to notice the gulf, and, paradoxically, student reactions to the readings were evidence of their own "listening."

In this particular week, students reflected upon Metzl and Hansen's structural competency [2], which ends with structural humility as a way to anticipate the limits of a structural approach to clinical engagement. The readings foregrounded the conundrum of addressing individual experiences of illness while attending to structures that enable or inhibit health-care access and delivery. Naming the acknowledgment of this conundrum humility, Metzl and Hansen argue that we must never presume a clinician, or medical educator for that matter, can ever possibly resolve the contradictions and tensions built in to this *individual cum structural* conundrum. The experience of illness and of providing care is always already both individually and structurally.

I have developed the approach to the paradox of this conundrum that I call *relational*. It is relational because it begins and ends with student self-awareness as it impacts their clinical encounters, with patient and other clinical professionals. It is political because I emphasize the work of relationship as an oft ignored but critically necessary process of simultaneously transforming clinical practice and the world. When physicians lack awareness of what their own conditioning brings to the clinical encounter, they easily label structural barriers to treatment as noncompliance or treatment avoidance.

Theoretical Framework: Relational Politics

In this case essay, I will explore just a few of the principles of this approach drawing special attention to the ways students can be accompanied through what is for many their first encounter with the often invisible paradox of self-other. Relational politics is the idea that not only are all things and people connected but that those connections are continuously renewed or weakened by the way we encounter one another and our world. Teachers of all kinds [3], activist scholar theorists [4, 5], philosophers, and social scientists [6–9], to highlight only a very few, point to the fact that since "nothing comes before the relations that created it" [10], including our own sense of self and other, that making our world anew must entail the work of relation building. The principles in this case are meant to give an encouraging provocation to stay with the discomforts of our interconnectedness. It is from that pause in the repeated present encounters with another that our world will be remade. First I will describe the program in which this work was developed; then I will describe some of the most common dynamics in the classroom that enable professor and students to dance with the paradox of relational politics. A few principles of relational politics will be introduced such that they might be experimented with in your own practices.

Teaching and Learning "Medicine"

The Program in Medical Education for the Latino Community (PRIME-LC) started in 2004 after nearly a decade of academic planning and legislative lobbying. Framed as medical education about and for the Latino community, the program consists of 90 h of supplemental seminars taught by medical social scientists. It includes coursework and rotations catered to clinical care for the Spanish-speaking medically underserved, a master's degree of the students' choosing, and the chance to be part of a small supportive cohort. Now in its 15th year, PRIME-LC is simplistically seen by outsiders as a robust "cultural" lesson for doctors who want to work with Spanish-speaking patients. It is true that students learn about the history, culture, and politics of medicine in Latin America and the USA. And, to avoid the deep grooves of cultural competence, the idea that improved medical care can come by simply improving clinicians' understanding Latino culture; I am careful to select readings that cannot be easily reduced to something Latino specific. Health inequity, like all social arrangements, is structural [11, 12]. In my courses, the underlying tension designed to create productive cognitive challenges is more powerful than the formal curricula, however. To wit, to address clinical inequity requires cultural humility [13, 14], clinical advocacy, and addressing the structural factors that account for disease and health-care inequities. But how does humility work to this end?

Humility is an interesting word. "The Other always lies beyond the self," notes Levinas passim [13]. I take this to mean, I am not you, you are not me. I am not my students and they are not their professors. Patients are not their doctors and doctors are not their patients. Pretty simple right? It does not mean self-abnegation or self-derision or self-diminishment. Rather, I argue, it requires *first and foremost a serious engagement with the self and not the other*. The basic premise of my work with students is that to change clinical inequity requires that medical students work on themselves as advocates and people as much as they work to alleviate the suffering of any given patient or fix a particular clinical protocol.

"Know Thyself, Nothing in Excess, Certainty Ruins." Readers may recognize these inscriptions of Delphi on the Sanctuary of Apollo on Mount Parnassus, Greece. In my work with medical students, I repeatedly return to the first edict, "Know Thyself." This is the foundation for the first rule for relational politics. By way of another illustration, I will describe my pedagogical use of Metzl and Hansen's 2013 article [2].

In a recent undergraduate class, a student approach me, a premed, who was about to go to a city in Guatemala on an exchange. I surmised that it was a community engagement and service learning exchange. We had been reading medical anthropology all quarter and she paused to ask herself, and then me, "What should I ask the people I work with in this village if I want to understand how or if homeless children access health care or what they do when they get sick?" I told her I have no idea but that the first question she should ask once she is there is what she just asked me. In doing this, I gave her what is one of the foundational principles of relational politics and community engagement. Ask real questions, those that reflect what you really need to know. However, this requires humility, perspective, trust, respect, and relational competency to begin with such a question. It also goes against the unidirectional grain of professional biomedicine where the physician knows the answers. And, in asking real questions, you are showing up as you are, not pretending to have an answer, and, as long as you are also ready to change the question altogether, you are primed for transforming the clinical encounter, learning a lot more than you thought possible and...having a greater impact.

This leads me to the second provocation of relational politics. Get out of your comfort zone. We must cross divides and bridge worlds if we are to engage with the world as it is. Too often, whether you are an educator, researcher, clinician, or advocate, we engage with a world of our own imagination, and then we get confused when the world pushes back [15] and doesn't conform to our fantasies. This is especially true for clinical, pedagogical, or research relationships with people who experience complex health and social problems. However, it is also true in all relationships. I learned this the only way such insight can be truly learned. A hard way, through trial and error, through struggling to practice my teaching and research activity in the most relationally honest way I could. Very much like all my relationships. By making mistakes, always trying to meet people where they are, and holding firm to my own structural humility practices in the classroom and beyond.

The Path: Listening to Communities

In the larger work from which this provocation is derived, I explore the connections between the epigenetic and the social lifeworlds I encounter in a place I call Central City [16]. Located less than an hour south of Los Angeles, Central City is one of the most diverse cities in the USA. Nearly 68% of residents live at or below 200% of the US federal poverty rate and contend with gentrification, overcrowding, and struggling schools. Central City is also home to an array of youth and adult residents, who, along with their institutional allies, enact their persistent creative leadership and love of community every day. I was asked to work with Central City residents after a leukemia scare in two elementary schools. PRIME students begin rotations in

Central City during the summer before their first year in medical school. In this inner city and distressed neighborhood, feeling unsafe from crime and law enforcement is the structural violence [17], and systemic unjust mistreatment residents have identified as the root cause of their poor health. By criminals in the streets, by NGO, and by city operatives, residents report being excluded, violated, and abused. This is why in my research as in my courses, I practice a deeply relational approach. Neighborhood residents, like patients and distressed medical students, do not need me to hammer away at them for their shortcomings, their ignorances, and their suffering. Who needs to be related to through that lens? Rather, I work to meet them and thus bring the self that I cultivate to their strengths, not their deficits. Strengths and asset-based

Graphic Box or Figure

Four keys to structural humility:

1. Ask real questions that recognize the expertise of "patients:" we all need help from others.
   Asking real questions means you recognize this truth. A doctor needs a patient's story. A researcher needs a research participant. As students we need good teachers. Collaborators need good partners. We all need good people in our lives, to wit, patients, MDs, students, partners, collaborators, and experiential experts of all kinds. A real question is one for which you do not already have an answer.
2. Discomfort is a good thing. Asking real questions should make us uncomfortable. We should get out of our comfort zones.
   Engaging with others as the experts of their own lives, by which I mean those closer to the object of our concern, requires humility. If we stay in our social, intellectual orbit, our emotional comfort zones, our worldviews, we will never actually meet people who can teach us lessons we may need to learn or hear the lessons from those with whom we already interact.
3. Know your place: Be someone you'd like to know. We all come from somewhere important.
   Knowing your place means doing your homework. Not only about the people and places you hope to encounter but also about yourself. After all, there are reasons you don't know what you don't know... and you should work to discover what those reasons are. Excellent clinicians acknowledge the limits of their knowledge and skill. Think how annoying people who think they know something are when they really don't. Also, it makes for poor clinical practice. This is the essence of structural humility.
4. People are *not* their problems. Imagine how it feels to be defined by your most obvious struggles. People may experience poverty, insecurity, or illness. However, a relationally competent person understands that we all experience challenges and that we all have creativity, intelligences, hopes, dreams, and talents that motivate and enable our daily lives.

approaches [18, 19] make the most sense because they counter the patronization and alienation anyone feels when they are treated as weak and incapable. It is far better to build on strengths than to further fixate on challenges.

Key Learnings: Accompaniment to a Deeper Structural Competence

In the preamble to the class on structural competence, I tell my students that we often hear about cultural competence, which in study after study we find is only a bit better than stereotyping. And there is no way we can learn enough stereotypes for every kind of difference that we might encounter. Structural competence, I argue, simply means understanding that you bring into any relationship a lifetime of experiences, resources, knowledges, and privileges that are not of your own making, but of the confluence of biography, biology, history, and institutional arrangements.

Relationally speaking, this means your relationship, your engagement with others, is always already structured by inequities and inequalities you yourself did not create. Medical students in my program are especially keen to be on the right side of this paradox. Much of class discussion, especially early in the course, before we know each other, are student rehearsals with each other and me of all the ways they are already socially conscious.

However as the course progresses, and those gaps in clinical settings reveal themselves, they start to see that wanting to be humble and good and on the right side of social justice does not make inequities go away; in fact it may accentuate structural differences and make relating across great social divides more difficult. "Know thyself" is about knowing your place, the preconditions that brought you to this room, with this patient, at this time in history, in this place.

So what's this have to do with Central City? After about a year of work with residents, I started to hear a word that intrigued me. The word was accompaniment/ acompañamiento. And it had something to do with the way people worked with one another to solve personal and community problems. And I have learned that accompaniment/acompañamiento is a practice and orientation that is as refined and nuanced as that practiced by any lab tech or experimentalist. It is when Elsa leads her first neighborhood meeting or Victor testifies to city council for the first time, and we support them before with encouragement, during with our affirming presence, and congratulate them on their courage and intelligent performances. It is when we celebrate with Josie when her A1C drops another two points, encouraging her to keep doing whatever she is doing and offering our help with anything in her life. Accompaniment, a Catholicism-inspired term made popular by the late Salvadoran archbishop Oscar Romero, means to join with another for a while, to show up fully, with our hearts and minds to create or to travel together where and how the path we make leads. It could be to solve a problem, to care for one another, or simply to experience life together for a while [20–22]. Of course it also has musical reference, to make music with someone together.

Acompañamiento/accompaniment is a good principle for clinical care, for research, for advocacy, and for relationships writ large. Because it also describes a way to compose life and to compose the practices of caring for another, it further compels us to consider that the life of patients and the life in the clinic are best considered together and not in the socially reproductive manner that their separation implies. My campus is 15 min from the inner city neighborhood whose people helped teach me these lessons. For many, those 15 min may as well be 100 miles. The social distance between the campus and the neighborhood is that vast. To know my place, to be structurally competent is to know that the two places are deeply connected historically, socially, physically, and in many other ways. Workers on my campus live in Central City, a place some of my colleagues and neighbors are afraid of. The restaurant I frequent is owned by a teacher whose family comes from a Central City. Or the park I most love came from the annexing of Native land long ago forcing them to lose their family home and move. All connected histories. Most of my medical students work in Central City as part of their clinical rotations. So, in the clinic and outside it, in my university and outside of it, here and there, us and them, accompaniment is a meditation on relationality par excellence, that is, how we treat and are treated by those with whom we encounter in all spaces of our life, not only those we designate as "research," or clinical, or professional. The personal … you see… is political.

Research and clinical relationships are not special, unique, or apart from all relationships we might have. This point underlies all the others. This becomes all the more apparent and important when status differentials, structural advantages, or privileges are obvious but also when they are not.[1]

Relational politics are central to clinical care because relationships have an embodied, biological impact on patients and communities. For example, what—I ask—are the metabolic indices of epigenetics, methyl groups and histones, dose responses temporally sensitive that trigger in a cell when flooded with stress hormones because we have been misunderstood and experience chronic hardship, police misconduct, workplace abuse, racism, or domestic or structural violence? What about when we are praised, feel safe, solve a problem, or experience the care of another or our own sense of power? How does THAT impact our bodies? Are we asking such questions, is our clinical care based upon them, and if not why not? As I write elsewhere, residents in the neighborhood where I learn know that poverty and police violence make them sick [16]. When residents were asked what makes them sick, they responded that they do not feel safe. They understand the principles of epigenetics if not the technical language.

---

[1] Relationships aren't just about people, though. Organizational theorists have shown that relationships are key for inclusion and for ways of getting things done because relationships shape who talks to who, what gets linked to what, and when (Quick and Feldman, 2011). This kind of relationality is not only between people but between issues, objects, and sequences of actions as well. Relationships are about connections of all kinds (Strathern, 2014). The implications of making these connections, health, knowledge, engagement, and relationality, are that equity and justice, fairness, and respectful treatment of all people—political as these may sound—can be practices in labs and clinical encounters of all kinds.

Perhaps this is why residents in Central City are quick to notice if someone is mindlessly advancing their own agenda at the expense of that of the group, of the person speaking, or the meeting at hand. For example, in one of my community consultant meetings, a shy young person, I will call her Melissa, spoke up for the first time in a meeting. I had convened the group to think aloud together about how meetings were being run. We had spent so many hours of meetings in the initiative and not a lot of time to reflect on them. Melissa came with her mother. When it was her turn, she said, "In my youth group, meetings are run like this. Cards are handed out so we take turns with different roles. Notetaker, facilitator, encourager, researcher, time keeper." I asked, "What's the encourager do?" She replied, "When someone says something, the encourager's job is to connect it to the conversation or come up afterword and let them know they were heard and ask if there's anything else they wanted to say." Nothing says "you are not caring for us" or "I don't matter" like showing up to a meeting and being ignored or having someone push their agenda. But what does it take to "show up" otherwise? What does "caring for us" mean? I submit to you that the answer to this question is as intimate as our closest relationships. How do we not show up with our agenda at the dinner table? When negotiating with a partner, aging parent, boss or child, student, professor, collaborator, or colleague? I think the answer is different for each of us. It entails equal parts biography, psychology, sociology, and richness of daily life and context. And it requires relational politics of the kind I am learning about and sharing with you here.

Final Relational Competence Principle: People Are *not* Their Problems

In Central City, my team and I have learned about listening, about designing processes that juggle outcomes (getting things done), and inclusion. At the end of the day, Central City residents seek connection, belonging, respect, and dignity, within the collaborative that my team and I accompany, as in their life writ large. These are not distinct sets of relationality. This is a crucial insight. And it is one I gained by watching closely resident leaders and by misunderstanding and being misunderstood. Relationships take work. But 10 min in places like Central City, with those relational experts, comrades, street corner mayors, and wise, passionate, steadfast, cautious but optimistic ones that make a place thrum, which keep it going in spite of the conditions, would likely collapse the market for antidepressants. Because that spirit, the respiriting that Grace Lee Boggs [5] writes about, is what keeps people in places like Central City, Detroit, Flint, New York, Atlanta from abject poverty of the soul. It's deep democracy (cite) to its core. The clinical questions, if we were to take this seriously, would be the following: Why are most people *not* diabetic, sickly, on drugs, or violent in these seemingly impossible conditions? What are those people doing? What might we learn from them? We miss these keys to making a better world by focusing only on the problems. Focusing on people's deficits, their hardships aren't respectful relationality.

Most of us would avoid a relationship if it required us to perform and rehearse our deepest personal and political challenges because that was all someone was interested in. However, that is exactly how clinical practice and the majority social science research can come across. Therefore, being humble deep listeners in the relational politics required for equitable lifeworlds requires that we be intentional, conscious, and transparent about the relational qualities of our work.

Applying Deep Listening and Accompaniment to Other Situations

Self-other, we-they, you-I, and us-them, these languages and behaviors of divisions are well analyzed by philosophers and those in the humanities and social sciences. It is part of the concept of humility that Tervalon and Murray-Garcia [14], Hunt [13], and Metzl and Hansen [2] draw our attention to. Unfortunately many well-meaning people and professionals who have made the civic or global engagement turn appeal to transactional ways of addressing these divisions or solving complicated problems [23]. You give me this and I will give you that. If you do this or that, I will give you what I have or what you want. Is this how you would treat people you respect, people you want to have long-lasting meaningful equitable relationship? People with whom you are making a better world? No. But this is old politics as usual and what stands for social action across old social divides. But in Central City, commitments to inclusion and accompaniment, as Melissa's youth meetings demonstrate, are being developed to transform the world one meeting and one initiative at a time through the WAY we do things and the way we treat one another. Melissa and her peers will always know when they are being disrespected, and they will always have a better way in their toolbox. I argue that it is time to apply those and dozens more relational insights to the clinic, the sciences, and politics writ large. In fact, I argue, it already is being applied, but our human service infrastructures are so structured around to people's problems that we fail to recognize it. Relational politics, as I imagine them, aspire to a most fundamental act of recognition. To wit, you and I are making together a world that has yet to become and neither of us will get to prefigure that world.

Medical students often want to know what to do in these troubled times having gained a glimpse of insight from the readings. They ask, how can they be a clinician otherwise? In my class I ask my students to think of all the ways they currently take care of other people, at work, at school, at home. To think about the little ways, they already deeply listen and make a difference in the lives of those people; some they love, some they just happen to know, and some just because. "Make a list," I tell them. THIS is where you begin. Build upon these relational skills, these politics. Make these people and these relationships your teachers for facing and addressing this troubled world and these seemingly impossible problems. I tell them that they already have the seeds of what they need and are already making a world otherwise, one relationship at a time, whether they like it or not, understand it or not, and in this way they are making the world anew. This is what is needed for us to see what works, to learn from another, and to make a better world. My daily question is, am I ready to engage and thereby become otherwise? Are you?

References

1. Montoya M. Making the Mexican diabetic: race, science, and the genetics of inequality. 1st ed. Berkley: University of California Press; 2011.
2. Metzl JM, Hansen H. Structural competency: theorizing a new medical engagement with stigma and inequality. Soc Sci Med. 2014;103:126–33.

3. hooks b. Teaching community: a pedagogy of hope. 1st ed. New York: Routledge; 2003.
4. Fischlin D, Heble A, Lipsitz G. The fierce urgency of now: improvisation, rights, and the ethics of cocreation. Durham: Duke University Press Books; 2013.
5. Boggs GL, Kurashige S, Glover D. The next American revolution: sustainable activism for the twenty-first century. First Edition, Updated and Expanded Edition, New Afterword with Immanuel Wallerstein edition. Berkeley: University of California Press; 2012.
6. Benjamin A. Towards a relational ontology: philosophy's other possibility. Reprint edition. Albany: State University of New York Press; 2016.
7. Emirbayer M. Manifesto for a relational sociology. Am J Sociol. 1997;103(2):281–317.
8. Haraway DJ. Staying with the trouble: making kin in the Chthulucene. 1st ed. Durham: Duke University Press Books; 2016.
9. Strathern M. Reading relations backwards. J R Anthropol Inst. 2014;20(1):3–19.
10. Escobar A. Thinking-feeling with the earth: territorial struggles and the ontological dimension of the epistemologies of the south. AIBR Rev Antropol Ib. 2016;11(1):11–32.
11. Williams DR, Mohammed SA. Racism and health II: a needed research agenda for effective interventions. Am Behav Sci. [Internet]. 2013;57(8). Available from: https://www.ncbi.nlm.nih.gov/pmc/articles/PMC3863360/
12. Krieger N. Why epidemiologists cannot afford to ignore poverty. Epidemiology. 2007;18(6):658–63.
13. Hunt LM. Beyond cultural competence: applying humility to clinical settings. The park ridge center. Bulletin. 2001;24:3–4.
14. Tervalon M, Murray-García J. Cultural humility versus cultural competence: a critical distinction in defining physician training outcomes in multicultural education. J Health Care Poor Underserved. 1998;9(2):117–25.
15. Barad K. Meeting the universe halfway: quantum physics and the entanglement of matter and meaning. Second Printing edition. Durham: Duke University Press Books; 2007.
16. Montoya MJ. Potential futures for a healthy city: community, knowledge, and hope for the sciences of life. Curr Anthropol. 2013;54(S7):S45–55.
17. Farmer P. On suffering and structural violence: a view from below. Daedalus. 1996;125(1):261–83.
18. Saleebey D. The strengths perspective in social work practice: extensions and cautions. Soc Work. 1996;41(3):296–305.
19. Whiting L, Kendall S, Wills W. An asset-based approach: an alternative health promotion strategy? Community Pract. 2012;85:25–8.
20. Romero O, Sobrino J, Martin-Baro I. Voice of the voiceless: the four pastoral letters and other statements. Maryknoll: Orbis Books; 1985.
21. Transcripts | Paul Farmer Discusses Accompaniment at Harvard's Kennedy School [Internet]. [cited 2018 Oct 3]. Available from: https://www.lessonsfromhaiti.org/press-and-media/transcripts/accompaniment-as-policy/
22. Lynd S. Accompanying: pathways to social change. Reprint ed. Oakland: PM Press; 2012.
23. Transactions Transformations Translations > PERE > USC Dana and David Dornsife College of Letters, Arts and Sciences [Internet]. [cited 2018 Oct 3]. Available from: http://dornsife.usc.edu/pere/metrics/

Allying with Our Neighbors to Teach Structural Competence: The Yale Department of Psychiatry Structural Competency Community Initiative (YSCCI)

Robert M. Rohrbaugh, Billy Bromage, John A. Encandela, Virginia T. Spell, Bridgett Williamson, and Walter S. Mathis

The Problem

In most psychiatry training programs, residents learn in depth about diagnosis of psychiatric illness, treatments like psychopharmacology and psychotherapy, and, if they are lucky, treatments like psychosocial rehabilitation that focus on helping patients with jobs and housing. While there is wide recognition that social inequalities result in physical and mental health disparities for segments of the US population [1], inclusion of information about health disparities and methods to address disparities is irregularly addressed in medical education [2]. Most programs have a minimal curriculum that focuses on cultural competency, but as Hansen and Metzl have pointed out, some things commonly interpreted as being based on culture might better be conceptualized as based on structural issues that patients face in their neighborhood [3]. While the emphasis of most residency training on diagnosis and treatment is important as these trainees will be asked to work in these modalities with patients, the Yale Department

R. M. Rohrbaugh (✉)
Department of Psychiatry, Office of International Medical Student Education, Yale School of Medicine, New Haven, CT, USA
e-mail: robert.rohrbaugh@yale.edu

B. Bromage · B. Williamson · W. S. Mathis
Department of Psychiatry, Yale School of Medicine, New Haven, CT, USA
e-mail: billy.bromage@yale.edu; Bridgett.williamson@yale.edu; walter.mathis@yale.edu

J. A. Encandela
Teaching and Learning Center, Yale School of Medicine, New Haven, CT, USA
e-mail: john.a.encandela@yale.edu

V. T. Spell
Urban League of Southern Connecticut, Stamford, CT, USA
e-mail: vtspell@ulsc.org

© Springer Nature Switzerland AG 2019
H. Hansen, J. M. Metzl (eds.), *Structural Competency in Mental Health and Medicine*, https://doi.org/10.1007/978-3-030-10525-9_13

of Psychiatry residency program leadership was convinced that residents also needed to understand the barriers patients faced when attempting to be healthy when implementing care plans in the community. Our challenge was helping psychiatry residents learn about the structures that are barriers to health in a neighborhood and to ask what might help individuals in the neighborhood overcome those barriers.

While we could teach about these issues in the classroom by giving a lecture about the different structures in the community and how they might impact patient lives, we felt that this would be unlikely to have much of an effect. Having a faculty member (who is not part of the communities where many of our patients live) teach about those neighborhoods also seemed problematic to us. We wondered how we could make knowledge about the neighborhood structures "sticky" so residents would be maximally impacted and how we could teach them about the neighborhoods through the eyes of community members living in the neighborhood.

In the first years of the Yale Structural Competency Curriculum Initiative (YSCCI), we had assigned small groups of residents to different neighborhoods, and they were asked to explore the neighborhoods of New Haven. The small groups of residents then made a presentation to the larger group. Many times, residents reported neighborhood statistics on joblessness and crime, but at times, residents had not interacted with any people living in the neighborhood to find out about how unemployment or crime affected them or to find out about programs to help them overcome these structural problems. Nothing was presented on what people living in the neighborhoods liked about the neighborhood. In the final year before we re-evaluated and added more components to the YSCCI, three residents reported driving through a neighborhood but said they were too frightened to get out of the car to talk with neighborhood residents. It seemed to us that our structural competency initiative might be reinforcing stereotypes about the neighborhoods of New Haven rather than teaching the residents about structural competency.

Theoretical Framework

In order to bring the perspective of individuals living in the neighborhoods, we invited a person living with mental illness who works as a peer mentor at our local community mental health center and a community leader to join our planning group. Their perspectives have been incredibly helpful as we made changes to the program. First, we decided to fundamentally change the education goal from one in which residents see the neighborhood through their eyes to one in which the residents learn about the neighborhoods through the perspectives of individuals living in the neighborhood. However, in order to do this, we needed to recruit more peer mentors and more community leaders from each neighborhood of New Haven that we would visit. This was made easier by working with a community organizer at the community mental health center; his connections with peers and with leaders in the community were critical to being able to organize this effort.

We also recognized that we were asking groups composed of peers, community leaders, and residents to talk about very difficult topics like poverty, race, segregation, and access to resources. These are topics that can be challenging to talk about in a group of individuals who know each other well, but could be especially challenging in a group which had just met and in which several power dynamics were at play including physician/patient and community leader/community member as well as power dynamics around differences in gender, race, and ethnicity. Based on an innovative approach first used by Yale medical students, we invited a member of the Yale Art Gallery into our planning group. In using prompts based on drawing exercises and art exhibits, we initially approached difficult topics in a less personal manner by asking them to analyze artwork that invokes concepts of race, class, colonialism, and contemporary social inequalities. Based on the suggestion of the community leader on the planning committee, we added a session to view and discuss a documentary about the displacement of low-income homeowners in a neighborhood that residents visit on the tours. The session includes a discussion led by community leaders from the neighborhood featured in the documentary to further nurture the exploration of difficult topics together.

The Path

A planning committee was convened to refine the structural competency training that would be required for all second-year psychiatry residents. Along with five psychiatry faculty members, the planning committee included a community leader, an individual working as a peer advocate, third- and fourth-year psychiatry residents, and faculty members to ensure representation of all stakeholders. The planning committee determined that the YSCCI would be a community immersive experience led by the peer advocates and community leaders with the specific aim of allowing the second-year residents to explore the influence neighborhood structures have on health and to understand community programs that could facilitate health. This included highlighting how resilience is nurtured in the neighborhoods, so that psychiatry residents do not perceive the communities simply as pathological. The five neighborhoods were selected based on demographic representation in the clinics/hospitals served by second-year residents. The SCI was implemented over three non-consecutive days in fall of 2016 and consisted of (1) an evening team building exercise at the University Art Gallery, (2) a day exploring the neighborhoods, and (3) a second-year resident presentation session.

Eighteen second-year psychiatry residents were randomly assigned to five groups—three to four residents for each of the five neighborhoods. Implementation of the YSCCI began at the Yale Art Gallery where residents and community members met for a brief discussion of the concept of structural competency. Each team was comprised of a community member who is a peer advocate, a community leader, and three to four residents. Also, each team was assigned a teaching fellow from the art gallery who helped team members became familiar with each other through an ice-breaking exercise in which dyads sat back to back, with one member describing an art object while another drawing it based on the description.

After this fun exercise, the teaching fellow led each group to an object that represented disparity in one manner or another. Examples of objects included a painting depicting a party of well-dressed people inside a well-appointed house while outside the house were individuals who are thin and poorly dressed and are burning wood in order to be protected against the cold winter night; a sculpture depicting a person who has passed out or died with a needle stuck in his arm; and an eighteenth-century painting showing a Rhode Island family displaying their favorite possessions including a black man with an iron ring around his neck. The first step in the discussion was each member of the group describing what they saw in order to begin to feel comfortable using language that describes disparities, consequences of disparities, and race of the individuals being depicted. Next, the groups were encouraged to discuss what they inferred was being depicted including the role that the history of racism has played in perpetuating disparities. This experience allowed team members to practice using language that would facilitate the discussions group members were likely to have with one another in the community.

To augment the experiences of the Art Gallery session, and at the suggestion of a community leader, a film component was added to the introductory portion of the YSCCI. In a separate session, 1 week after the Art Gallery session, residents, peer advocates, and community leaders, including both those leading tours and other invited leaders, viewed a documentary film chronicling New Haven homeowners fighting to save their homes from demolition. The film follows a group of homeowners and community organizers, faith leaders, urban designers, and lawyers who worked with the homeowners to develop a campaign to resist building a school where their homes stood. The film is set in one of the neighborhoods in which tours happen during the YSCCI. The film touches on themes related to structural factors including racism, power asymmetries in city planning and breaking up low-income communities, the legacy of urban renewal, and access and lack of access to official channels of power. During the discussion that followed the film, residents had an opportunity to ask questions about the themes, share their insights, and participate with community leaders and peer advocates in a general discussion. Some of the community leaders facilitating the post-film discussion were involved in the struggle portrayed in the film, which added depth to the conversation. Similar to the Art Gallery session, the viewing and discussion provided a safe and structured yet engaging and sometimes raw forum for residents to discuss difficult topics with the people who would lead them through their neighborhoods in the subsequent session.

In the second component of the YSCCI, the small groups went out into the neighborhoods of New Haven where community members led them along a route with prearranged stops, as well as spontaneous opportunities to observe situations that presented themselves, in one of the five neighborhoods. Two of the neighborhoods had a primarily African-American population. The third had a primarily Latino population, a significant portion of which was undocumented. The fourth had a primarily African-American and Caucasian population. The fifth had a primarily African-American and Latino population, but had experienced a recent influx of refugees from Afghanistan and Syria. All five neighborhoods were made up of primarily low-income households. Community members narrated the tour with their own experiences in the neighborhood; these narratives differed somewhat depending on the perspective of whether the narrator was a community leader or a peer facilitator. Residents were exposed to the education system and schools, housing conditions, community police substations, food stores, libraries, social welfare programs, and community gardens to demonstrate both the challenges to having a healthy life in the community and programs and community responses which can facilitate this process.

At noon, the tour leaders stopped outside a corner store and gave each participant an envelope that contained $2.00, which is the average amount that an individual on SNAP receives per meal in New Haven. Residents were told to go into the corner store and use their payment to buy a healthy lunch. Groups differed on how they attempted to meet this challenge. Most pooled their resources and still had difficulty finding healthy items to purchase, with many groups sharing sandwiches made with processed meats or peanut butter. Others who did not pool their resources selected a bottle of water and a small bag of nuts or chips.

The experiential nature of the YSCCI allowed for teachable moments that would be outside the experience that could be developed in the classroom. Residents who complained about the distances travelled by foot on a hot day or the wait for the bus were reminded that these were the ways that their patients travelled for their treatment. Residents who took the bus were late in returning because the bus ran late even though they were at the bus stop at the appointed time. Privilege was discussed in the context of a corner store owner, who is known to be hostile to the community, but who gladly provided a free lunch to the group once he heard that they were Yale residents. One issue that was especially upsetting to the residents was hearing a relatively unvarnished account of community members' experiences with and attitudes toward Yale University and the Yale New Haven Hospital. Although we have a diverse residency class, most have identified to some extent with Yale, and it was challenging for them to hear these negative accounts about Yale having displaced people from their homes as it expanded and about their experiences as neighbors to a wealthy institution that they feel does little to improve their lives.

In the next component of the YSCCI, members of the small group discussed what they thought had been most compelling about the neighborhood visit. Residents then developed a short 10-min PowerPoint presentation that discussed the particular structural issues that the group felt had been most compelling through photographs taken during the neighborhood visit. Residents incorporated a brief reference to an academic perspective on that issue based on short articles and podcasts that were provided by YSCCI leaders. The YSCCI planning group hoped these presentations would ensure that the larger group was educated about other neighborhoods, about other resources, and about other structural issues than the one they had investigated. A panel of community advocates and faculty invested in public psychiatry critiqued the presentations and added another perspective, often historical, to the resident presentations.

Outcomes of the YSCCI were determined through listening to conversations after group members returned from the neighborhood visit and listening to the presentations and by a series of three focus groups. These post-seminar feedback focus groups were held in separate 1-h sessions with each stakeholder group: second-year residents, peer advocates, and community leaders. An objective and experienced focus group moderator, who was not part of planning or implementing the YSCCI, developed a feedback group protocol with planning committee members. Similar questions were developed for the three groups, with slight modifications to best represent the role of group members in the overall initiative. Participants were primarily asked to give perceptions of effective and less-than-effective components of the 3-day seminar, as well as overall recommendations for future iterations of the initiative. The focus groups were deemed exempt by the university's institutional review board.

After informed consent was given by participants, a rapid assessment approach [4] was used to take notes in place of audio recording, which was thought to be a potential inhibitor of frank conversation especially among second-year residents and peer advocates [5]. To assure validity, a summary of themes discussed in each component of the group process was offered by the moderator, and participants had the opportunity to modify or add to the summary points.

After each feedback meeting, notes were coded and codes were organized into themes and stakeholder recommendations. Themes and recommendations were compared and contrasted across stakeholder groups. After arriving at a final list of key themes and findings for each group, this summary was sent by email to participants with a request for revisions of further feedback. Members of all three groups agreed on lists of themes and findings without further revision. This final step provided an additional validity check on findings.

Key Learnings

Among the three focus groups—one focus group with residents, one with peers, and one with community leaders—all reported that the experience was compelling and made them think more about the community structures that were sometimes invisible even to individuals living in the community. All groups felt they had learned about barriers to health in the community and, importantly, seeing evidence of community resilience through community gardening and community watch programs as well as government-supported programs like libraries and job resource centers and NGO-supported programs like psychosocial rehabilitation centers for individuals living with mental illness in the community. Residents learned about Catholic Worker houses, where a family agreed to house, feed, and clothe individuals who needed help. Residents met police officers who seemed to genuinely care about the community, while other groups met police officers who seemed quite disparaging of the community they were assigned to serve. Residents reported having to take public transportation or walking would make them think twice about the reasons why a patient might be late for an appointment. While community members believed the SNAP lunch experience was an important learning experience for the residents, some residents thought it was an inadequate attempt to provide them with an experience of poverty. Residents felt defensive during the YSCCI when hearing negative comments about Yale from community members and from the panel, and residents also felt they needed to protect the community by emphasizing the positive aspects of the community when making their presentations. While residents liked the YSCCI experience overall, many thought it still left them feeling disconnected from the community. Consistent with this view, residents did not find the presentations to be useful and wondered whether working on a community resource guide with community members might be a better capstone experience. Several also reported interest in following up with specific programs they had visited to develop deeper community ties. To address this feedback, a subgroup of the planning committee has been formed to determine an effective activity, including clearly stated learning objectives, to elicit PGY-2 residents' reflections about their experiences during the neighborhood tours, to tie those experiences to structural factors, and to begin to bridge these insights into clinical formulations. An exercise developed by the subgroup that will be used in the future asks each group of residents to compose a clinical vignette of a hypothetical patient from the neighborhood they have just toured, highlighting structural challenges and resources and how these are impacting the patient's physical and mental health and health care.

Stakeholders' feedback indicates that the execution of the seminar's goals can improve by clearly stating the objectives of the various components. For example, we will be clearer about the goal of the SNAP lunch experience; it was designed to illustrate food insecurity and the challenges of finding healthy food, not as an experience of poverty. We continue to believe the SNAP lunch exercise creates an invaluable opportunity for residents to experience in real time the multifaceted challenges of food insecurity—a knowledge that cannot be appreciated from reading neighborhood statistics. While community leaders and peer advocates felt empowered by its inclusion in the YSCCI, PGY-2 residents were unable to connect the exercise to clinical practicalities. This discordant feedback illustrates the need to improve the communication of the goals of the experience. Therefore, future iterations of the seminar will preface this experience with explicit instructions that illustrate the meaning and goals of such an exercise while maintaining an environment for open discussion of the experience among all stakeholders. Additionally, the experiential SNAP activity will be made more clinically relevant by coupling it with teaching second-year residents to use a two-question food insecurity screening questions to use during interviews [6]. Similarly, the objectives of the presentations were identified as unclear by stakeholders. Stakeholders indicated that the presentations were further complicated by the inclusion of community panelist who were not clear on their roles as co-educators.

The YSCCI provoked awareness of privileges as well as class consciousness in the PGY-2 residents. Community members gave straightforward reactions to the university and university hospital regarding, for example, their expansion into neighborhoods and resulting displacement of community members. This feedback was uncomfortable for residents to hear but highlights the transformative experience of assuming a position of power as a psychiatry resident and facilitating care in a community where negative feelings about institutions are prevalent. We feel it is important for PGY-2 residents to understand the significant dynamics between patient, community, and institution. Medical institutions have complicated histories with their surrounding neighborhoods [7]. For this reason, it is essential for psychiatry residents to gain knowledge of these histories, their potential impacts on access to care, and the feelings that their patients harbor toward the institutions they represent.

We have been imbedding the YSCCI in a new social justice and health equity-based curriculum that aims to ensure that psychiatry residents understand the origins of health disparities and how to avoid becoming the next generation of physicians contributing to these disparities. In addition to the YSCCI, psychiatry residents are trained to understand their own implicit biases and microaggressions, to develop person-centered treatment approaches, and to advocate at the individual, institutional, and policy system levels. The process of developing the YSCCI has provided us with the opportunity to partner with our patients and community members to teach our trainees. The outcome of this collaboration has been a more complex understanding of structures in our community and of our shared history, as well as the challenges that exist in implementing shared decision-making and advocacy efforts. We have begun to collaborate with the community in other aspects of our health equity and social justice curriculum.

While we strongly believe that the YSCCI was successful in teaching residents about community structures, there are several important limitations for others considering whether to implement a similar program. First, while the program emphasizes understanding neighborhood structures from a community perspective, residents are not taught nor do they practice how to employ this knowledge in patient care setting. We plan to expand the scope of the YSCCI to include this important element in future iterations of the program. For example, in the current iteration of the initiative, we are adding a facilitated reflection session with residents that asks them to contemplate lessons learned from the total experience of the components and to consider applications of these to interactions with their patients. Second, the program is resource intensive in both planning and implementation. The planning group meets for several months before implementation and then intensively when the YSCCI is being implemented. Collaborations with community partners and, for us, the Art Gallery are critical components of the program. Providing light meals facilitates the experience at the Art Gallery, on the neighborhood visit day and on the presentations day. Last, because this content and experiential learning model can be challenging, ample curricular time needs to be allocated to orient residents to the task and learning objectives and to reflection activities after the neighborhood visit.

References

1. Centers for Disease Control and Prevention. CDC health disparities & inequalities report—United States, 2013. MMWR. 2013;62(Suppl 3):1–87.
2. Westerhaus M, Finnegan A, Haidar M, Kleinman A, Mukherjee J, Farmer P. The necessity of social medicine in medical education. Acad Med. 2015;90(5):565–8.
3. Metzl JM, Hansen H. Structural competency: theorizing a new medical engagement with stigma and inequality. Soc Sci Med. 2014;103:126–33.
4. Compton MT. The social determinants of mental health. 1st ed. Shim RS, editors. Washington, DC: American Psychiatric Publishing; 2015.
5. Trotter RT, Needle RH, Goosby E, Bates C, Singer M. A methodological model for rapid assessment, response, and evaluation: the RARE program in public health. Field Methods. 2001;13(2):137–59.
6. Schroeder C, Neil RM. Focus groups: a humanistic means of evaluating an HIV/AIDS programme based on caring theory. J Clin Nurs. 1992;1(5):265–74.
7. Martin DG. Reconstructing urban politics: neighborhood activism in land-use change. Urban Aff Rev. 2004;39(5):589–612.

Community Health Workers as Accelerators of Community Engagement and Structural Competency in Health

Chau Trinh-Shevrin, MD Taher, and Nadia Islam

The Problem

The Model Minority Myth and Health Disparities Among Asian Americans: Chau Trinh-Shevrin, DrPH

As a Vietnamese refugee who came to the United States in the 1970s, I experienced firsthand the cultural, linguistic, and social barriers that Asian Americans face in navigating the healthcare system. The trauma associated with war, migration, and social isolation, as well as cultural differences and language barriers, made it challenging for my parents in seeking preventive and timely healthcare services. Similarly, providers at that time also had poor understanding of the stress and mental health concerns associated with migration and displacement and how that manifested in health outcomes. These issues were complicated in miscommunication due to language differences and misconceptions of the experience of pain or symptoms among their Asian American patients. Decades later, I learned from my research that my family's experience was not unusual: doctors are less likely to follow evidence-based guidelines and meet standards of care with their Asian American patients compared with other racial groups in preventing and managing chronic conditions [1–6]. I also learned that times have not changed dramatically in the care of Asian American patients even though there is increasing recognition that Asian Americans face just as many health challenges, including an increasing rate of diabetes and certain cancers. This neglect seems to be linked to the "model minority" stereotype of Asian Americans, promoted in American culture and media, which portrays them as uniformly hardworking, affluent, and healthy. Yet, Asian Americans are not all alike. There are substantial differences in language,

C. Trinh-Shevrin (✉) · MD Taher · N. Islam
Department of Population Health, NYU School of Medicine, New York, NY, USA

© Springer Nature Switzerland AG 2019

H. Hansen, J. M. Metzl (eds.), *Structural Competency in Mental Health and Medicine*,
https://doi.org/10.1007/978-3-030-10525-9_14

migration, and social experiences across Asian subgroups whose ancestral heritages hail from East, South, and Southeast Asia, and health concerns and risks vary across and within these communities [6].

The model minority misconception systemically influences how doctors and nurses provide healthcare to Asian Americans. In fact, the evidence suggests that aggregated data mask important differences – such as diet and health risks – that may affect health outcomes among more than 30 Asian ethnic subgroups. For example, diabetes rates are strikingly high for South Asians and Filipinos [3]. More than one in three individuals of South Asian and Filipino descent have diabetes [3], a rate that is substantially greater than for all other racial/ethnic groups.

A key goal of the NYU Center for the Study of Asian American Health (CSAAH) is to dispel the myth that Asian Americans are a model minority and the misperception that they do not face health challenges. In fact, among racial and ethnic minority populations in the United States, immigrant communities face a number of social and cultural challenges in health promotion and disease prevention, and Asian Americans are no exception. Asian Americans are the fastest growing minority group in the United States, estimated to increase to about 39 million people by 2060 – approximately 9.3% of the US population [7]. The American Community Survey (ACS) 2015 reported that nationally over 60% of Asian Americans are foreign born and more than 30% have limited English proficiency (LEP) [8], which can limit health and preventive care access and impair patient-provider communication [9–11]. The largest Asian American population in a US city is in New York City (NYC) [12]; approximately 1.2 million Asian Americans comprise 14.1% of the city's population with Chinese, South Asian, and Korean subgroups representing the largest NYC Asian subgroups [13].

Asian Americans in NYC face many dimensions of social disadvantage. For example, the poverty rate among Asian Americans in NYC is the highest compared to all other racial and ethnic groups. According to the NYC Office of the Mayor, the poverty rate in 2014 among Asian Americans was 27%, compared to white (14%), black (22%), and Latino (24%) populations; poverty rates are also rising the fastest among Asian Americans compared to all other groups [14]. One in four Asian Americans is living in poverty [14], and about 25% of Asian Americans have not graduated from high school [8]. Socioeconomic disparities are even more acute by subgroup. For example, the Bangladeshi population, the fastest growing Asian subgroup in NYC, experience a high rate of limited English proficiency when compared to other subgroups; about 53% of the NYC Bangladeshis speak English less than "very well" as compared with the citywide limited English proficiency (LEP) rate of 23% [15, 16]. NYC Bangladeshis are among the poorest of the Asian subgroups; approximately 33% of Bangladeshis in NYC live below the poverty line as compared with the citywide rate of 20%. NYC Bangladeshis also have lower high school completion and annual household income compared to citywide numbers [15].

There is a substantial body of evidence – much of which we have helped to build through our research efforts – that demonstrates that Asian Americans are disproportionately impacted by chronic diseases, with meaningful variation in risk and prevalence across subgroups [17–19], for example, diabetes disparities are striking for Asian Americans in the aggregate and in particular for South Asians and Filipinos with nearly one in three at risk [3]. Yet, they are often disconnected from healthcare institutions and further isolated by social distance due to their migration status, differences in language and cultural expectations, as well as lack of trust in health professionals.

Theoretical Framework

Community Health Workers, An Evidence-Based Approach to Reducing Diabetes Disparities

To reduce health disparities in minority and immigrant populations, there is a genuine need to build social and human capital and community leadership within these communities. The community health worker (CHW) model represents a compelling and powerful way to support the cultural, social, and health needs of underserved communities confronted with substantial barriers to accessing and navigating the healthcare system and understanding of the recommended guidelines for chronic disease prevention. CHWs are frontline health workers who are indigenous to the community in which they work. They understand the strength, value, and culture of the community members and speak their language. They are trusted members of the community and can easily build personal connections. They can engage local communities in health initiatives, which build capacity in the community, and CHWs take natural leadership in that process. CHWs build social networks and friendships and promote bonding among the community members.

As they are effective in many areas, CHWs are particularly useful in community-based participatory research (CBPR). CBPR promotes collaboration between community stakeholders and academic researchers, facilitates co-learning, ensures cultural appropriateness, and engages and empowers community members [16]. Integrating CHWs in CBPR can be instrumental to the success of a research project. CHWs accelerate community engagement strategies through research design, implementation, and dissemination of research findings to broader communities. CHWs are often more effective in outreach, recruitment, and retaining hard-to-reach communities confronted with substantial language and cultural barriers. CHWs also inform the development of targeted, tailored health messages and strategies that are both meaningful to the target communities and likely to be successful in supporting healthy behavior change. CHWs bridge the gap between patients and providers by serving as linguistic and cultural interpreters. For providers who face difficulties communicating with the patients or the patients who face language and cultural barriers, CHWs can play a vital role to bridge those gaps.

To illustrate the power and potential of CHWs as accelerators of community engagement and structural competency in health, we present the below perspectives of Dr. Nadia Islam, director of the DREAM (*D*iabetes *R*esearch *E*ducation and *A*ction for *M*inorities) Project and Mr. MD Taher, a DREAM CHW.

The Path

A Clinical Trial of Community Health Workers for Diabetes Care: Nadia Islam, PhD

"Why are so many aunties and uncles dying in our community?"

As a second-generation Bangladeshi immigrant, my community social network was critical to providing support and meaning for my identity in the United States. Though I have a large extended family, my parents left most of their family behind when immigrating to the United States in the 1970s, building a life for themselves largely without the emotional and instrumental support that relatives can provide. As such, making connections to other Bangladeshi and South Asian community members through cultural and religious events and gatherings at home and at shared community spaces like ethnic grocery stores and restaurants facilitated the creation of a second extended family for me in the United States. Growing up, these "aunties" and "uncles" were key figures in my life, celebrating birthdays, graduations, and other key milestones with us. As such, death and illness that were faced by these community members took on personal meaning, and as I grew up, our community was faced again and again by the early deaths of aunties and uncles through heart attacks, strokes, and complications of diabetes. In the already perplexing life of a teenager, these deaths did not make sense to me. My personal connection to these community tragedies compelled me to pursue public health and better understand what was happening in South Asian immigrant communities like mine. As a doctoral student at Columbia University, I immersed myself in literature and coursework on health disparities and conceptual frameworks for understanding what drives health inequities, but I was surprised that the voices of my own community were often absent in the literature – in fact, the research I found characterized Asian Americans as having better health than the rest of the population (at best) or (at worst) did not include data on Asian Americans at all.

I was fortunate to meet Dr. Trinh-Shevrin, another Asian American immigrant, during my graduate studies. Like me, Dr. Trinh-Shevrin was alarmed by the gap in our scientific and conceptual understanding of the health of Asian Americans and successfully established an NIH-funded research center, the NYU Center for the Study of Asian American Health, dedicated to understanding and addressing health disparities in the Asian American population in 2003. I began working with Dr. Trinh-Shevrin shortly after the Center was established and used the opportunity to directly tackle the problem of diabetes that had plagued my community for so many years.

Building on my personal experience that social networks are critical in immigrant communities like the Bangladeshi population, I worked with a community-based coalition to establish the DREAM (Project in 2007). The overall goal of the DREAM Project is to develop, implement, and test the efficacy of a CHW intervention designed to improve type 2 diabetes mellitus (T2DM) control and management in the Bangladeshi community of New York City. The strength and value of the DREAM Project in advancing structural competency is drawn directly from the CHWs themselves, and, as such, I realized that recruiting individuals who were respected and trusted leaders in the community was critical. During the early stages of the development of the project, CHWs with backgrounds in immigrant and student organizing and active in cultural and social efforts in the NYC Bangladeshi population were engaged. Similarly, the study established a community advisory board consisting of representatives from community and clinical settings that served the Bangladeshi community to ensure iterative feedback from stakeholders at every stage of the project implementation and evaluation.

The DREAM Project utilized a two-arm randomized control-trial design. Participants meeting eligibility criteria are recruited from community and clinical settings and randomized to either the treatment or control arm. Those in the treatment arm receive five group-based culturally and linguistically tailored educational sessions from a CHW and two one-on-one visits from the CHW to develop individualized goal-setting and health coaching. Intervention outcomes were assessed by tracking changes in clinical outcomes from baseline to completion of the project at 6 months; in addition, surveys were collected from participants to understand the impact of the program on health behavior change to support diabetes management, self-efficacy, and social support.

In the DREAM Project, CHWs served as a vital source of community knowledge and are closely involved in all aspects of the study, including the development of study instruments, data collection, informing research design, and interpreting study results. In addition, CHWs are involved in the dissemination of the intervention through community forums and ethnic media. In addition to reporting results of the intervention back to the community, community forums are also conducted in response to the community's concerns and questions regarding new policies and initiatives (e.g., Patient Protection and Affordable Care Act – ACA). These community forums facilitate co-learning among academic and community partners. Moreover, as the CHWs are fully involved in the project, it gives ownership of the project to the CHWs and the community they represent. Consequently, this practice builds capacity in the community by empowering CHWs and community members.

CHWs are effective interventionists and natural leaders. In order to be effective in their roles for the DREAM Project, each CHW completed an extensive training in a variety of skill sets and learning areas related to their various functions. Trainings included CHW history and adult learning, learning style and behavioral change, communication, informal counseling, group facilitation, chronic disease, and nutrition review. CHWs participated in trainings on an ongoing basis based on the availability of useful trainings as well as their expressed interest in content areas. In addition to CHW-specific trainings, each DREAM CHWs received extensive trainings on diabetes management skills. After receiving these trainings, CHWs effectively led the intervention sessions.

Community Health Worker Perspective: MD Taher, MPH of the DREAM Project

I was born in a rural area of Bangladesh. With nine siblings, I am the eighth child of my parents. Both of my parents had diabetes and died prematurely. My mother passed away in her early 50s. All my siblings now have diabetes, and within a period of 3 months this past year, two of my siblings passed away in Bangladesh. Diabetes is highly present in my family, and it is widely common for most of the families in Bangladesh. In addition to my parents and siblings, my uncles and aunts from maternal and paternal sides died from diabetes. Diabetes has tangled my family like tentacles of an octopus. I have witnessed and known many Bangladeshis in Bangladesh who suffer and die from diabetes. It is so profoundly common and insidious.

It has been almost 11 years since I came to the United States at the age of 22. I was naturally compelled to build connections to other members of my community as a new immigrant, becoming active in student groups and establishing a cricket league in New York City, helping to bring together young Bangladeshi immigrants like myself. I became involved with CSAAH through an internship with the DREAM Project while I was attending college. There, I had the opportunity to work with the DREAM CHWs who provided diabetes management skills to the Bangladeshis living in New York City. I felt a personal connection to work in a diabetes management project since many of my family members, including my loving mother and father, died due to the high burden of the disease in my community. I was only a boy of 13 when my mother died. After the internship, I accepted a position as a DREAM CHW. As an immigrant to the United States and through my work with the local Bangladeshi community, I found that diabetes is similarly as highly prevalent among the community members. I devoted myself to improve the skills and knowledge of diabetes and other chronic illnesses among my community members. At first, few people knew me. But after working with the community as a CHW, many people now know me. They listen to me and follow me; see me as a role model. I found myself easily accepted to my community as we have the same language, culture, and country of origin. By working as a CHW, I quietly developed leadership skills to mobilize community members to take ownership of their own health. I feel honored and blessed to work for the health of my community.

As a CHW serving Asian American immigrants, I realized the vital importance and effectiveness of building capacity and leadership within the communities to both improve population health and reduce chronic disease disparities. I have worked closely with the New York City Bangladeshi and South Asian communities, including Pakistani, Indian, and Nepali populations. One of the major challenges these communities face is the language barrier. I have seen the newer immigrants (those in the country living less than 5 years) struggling to make appointments with their doctors or understanding their doctors due to limited or no English proficiency. Many immigrants faced difficulties navigating the unfamiliar and complex healthcare system. These communities also lack culturally and linguistically tailored health education materials available for them. At times, they cannot comprehend important health information as they are in English and not culturally relevant for them. When Affordable Care Act (ACA) first started, many community members had no idea how to navigate the unfamiliar process. Women from these communities often rely on family members to bring them to health providers due to cultural reasons or lack of knowledge of how to navigate the large public transportation system. To mitigate those challenges, a CHW like myself plays a vital role. As a

CHW, I take on multiple roles including engaging local communities in health initiatives; bringing in individuals who are unfamiliar to the healthcare system; providing cultural linkages; contributing to building the patient-provider communication, patient and community education, and counseling; and enhancing adherence to care. To support my role and responsibilities, I participated in many trainings for the DREAM Project. These trainings increased my confidence and capacity. They were vital in helping me be effective in delivering the right messages in the right way that would encourage and activate change for supporting diabetes prevention and control. To further support my work, there were ongoing quality assurance and fidelity checks [20] and, when needed, discussions to debrief on specific cases and emerging challenges and tailored trainings to strengthen and deepen my health education capacity. The trainings and ongoing support and supervision empowered me in many ways.

While working as a CHW with the Bangladeshi community, I was able to take health initiatives to the community members who trusted me. They participated with great enthusiasm in those initiatives. I spoke their language; I understood their culture and values. I provided health information in their own language. Over the years, I have provided chronic disease management trainings, education, and counseling to community members. I shared my life experiences with them, which enhanced the level of trust. Moreover, I provided a platform for community members to build social networks by bringing them together to participate in these health initiatives. Group health events supported ways to engage community members and foster social capital. As a CHW facilitating events and discussions with various perspectives of community members and stakeholders, these community health engagement activities made me become a more effective leader of my community, I feel empowered and confident to effectively mobilize families and community for disease prevention and health promotion. While working as a CHW in DREAM Project, I felt that an MPH degree in community health would enhance my knowledge of program development and evaluation and prepare myself to better serve the community. I was very fortunate that DREAM Project thoroughly supported me in applying, attending, and achieving an MPH degree from New York University with a concentration in Community and International Health.

I assisted community members who had no English proficiency by going with them during their doctors' visits. This benefitted not only the patients but also the providers. I have also seen my female CHW colleague educate and show female community members how to navigate the subway system so that they could go to doctors' visits by themselves. Some of those women have never taken subway trains alone nor visited doctors alone. Prior to meeting their CHW, their family members used to accompany them during the visits, and family members feared that they would get lost if they traveled alone. After the trainings, those female community members were able to visit their doctors alone at the hospital. They felt confident and empowered. Yet, there remained the language barrier; but the presence of a CHW at the doctor's appointment eliminated that. In one particular instance, a community member requested me to accompany him on his doctor's visit. In previous meetings, the doctor and the patient could not communicate well with each other due to language barriers. My presence at the appointment was very useful for both the doctor and the patient – the doctor was able to relay important information regarding changes to the patient's medication regimen and worked with me to provide culturally tailored self-management advice related to diet and exercise to the patient. Within 3 months, the patient showed noticeable improvements in his diabetes management. In fact, the physician relayed that my work, as a CHW, in linking the gap in care for this patient contributed directly to his improved health outcomes. Another noticeable factor was that the providers had very little knowledge of South Asian culture in terms of foods and religious practices. My CHW colleagues and I organized cultural competency trainings on South Asian culture for the students, residents, and providers. These trainings were beneficial for providers as they increased their clinical capacity. And of course, CHWs were at the forefront of the trainings taking the ownership and leadership of these trainings. The doctors remarked that the information CHWs shared helped them provide more effective treatment to their South Asian patients.

As a CHW in DREAM Project, my services to the community members were not just limited to physical health. I have seen community members struggling with poverty. There was not enough money to buy foods; houses were crowded. They could not afford to rent houses with enough rooms. There were issues related to immigration status, domestic violence, mental illnesses, insurance access, racism, and cultural discrimination. Due to lack of appropriate documents, I have seen participants become severely depressed because they could not return to their country of birth, where they left their beloved children and family members more than 20 years ago. In addition, as they are undocumented, they could not get health insurance coverage to get necessary healthcare. As much as we could, my CHW colleagues and I helped community members apply for public housing and food stamps and connected them with appropriate resources for other social services they needed. These services promoted their health and well-being.

There are tough challenges related to being a CHW. I recognize how fortunate I am to have this position, to be part of CSAAH in supporting health promotion and disease prevention efforts. I also know that these roles are limited. While there is increasing recognition of the value of CHWs in healthcare systems and in population health strategies, there are many barriers to supporting full integration of CHWs. My CHW colleagues are constantly struggling to find positions in the traditional healthcare systems and clinical settings. Often I see challenges stemming from lack of understanding from other healthcare professionals around the role and functions of CHWs. At the community level, a key challenge is being able to balance working with clients on individual behavior change with creating and sustaining change at the interpersonal and neighborhood level. At the policy level, I also see that with the change in political administration, many in my community are deeply concerned about their social position, where they can turn to for assistance, and when they can seek care, which in turn influence both social and health disparities. Furthermore, given that many CHW programs are supported through healthcare reform efforts, there is uncertainty regarding the future of sustainable mechanism and career paths for this workforce.

Lessons Learned by the Authors

There were many indicators of effectiveness for the DREAM Project. Those who participated in the diabetes management program showed increased physical activity level, increased knowledge of diabetes, increased consumption of healthier foods, and improved blood pressure and cholesterol levels. In addition, a greater proportion of those who participated in the intervention achieved diabetes control compared to those who were in the control group. The greatest improvement occurred among individuals with uncontrolled diabetes (blood glucose levels of A1c $\geq$ 8) at baseline: among intervention participants with baseline A1c $\geq$ 8, mean A1c decreased by 0.7 ($p = 0.015$), while among control participants with a baseline A1c $\geq$ 8, mean A1c decreased by 0.2 ($p = 0.396$); the adjusted intervention effect among individuals with baseline A1c $\geq$ 8 was −0.5 ($p = 0.117$). The intervention group was significantly more likely to demonstrate a decrease in A1c at 6-month follow-up compared to the control group (55.2% vs. 42.5%, $p = 0.035$). Beyond clinical and behavioral outcomes, our intervention had a major impact on enhancing self-efficacy related to engaging in physical activity, healthy eating, and the ability to more effectively communicate with their physician. Participants who received the intervention were also more likely to report enhanced social support and trust in their friends and neighbors. Finally, we also engaged participants to facilitate our understanding of how they felt the program helped them make changes in their health, and through this we have identified key mechanisms through which CHWs can affect change with community members [21–23]. With the right balance of training and guidance, CHWs in the project brought about positive changes in health for community members. CHWs helped community members become active participants in their own health. CHWs and the participants also involved participants' friends and family members in the process of change for better health.

Through our collective efforts, representing nuanced and complementary perspectives, we have learned that CHWs can be effective leaders and change agents in empowering individuals and families to prioritize health, developing meaningful solutions for healthful behavior change, and mobilizing communities to improving access to care and health promotion efforts. CHWs have an immense potential to be leaders in the community and healthcare system if they are properly trained and guided.

- Effective CHWs by characteristic are natural leaders in their community, mobilizing and advocating for social justice and health equity. To further support leadership in community health promotion and disease prevention, CHWs should receive a wide range of instruction, such as mental health and motivational interview trainings that would address the other needs that are often presented by community members and can support focused discussions on disease management and wellness. These trainings will make them competent to work more effectively and efficiently with community members.
- Similarly, with the right balance of trainings and guidance, CHWs can complement and support the work of physicians, nurses, social workers, and other mem-

bers of the healthcare team. Many CHWs do not have high educational credentials, thus training that rigorously provide and utilize adult learning techniques are important to help support CHWs' capacity to successfully carry out necessary activities. It is also important that other members of the healthcare team have a clear understanding of CHW roles and responsibilities. In our own experience, we have seen how CHWs have advanced structural competency in different healthcare settings, from small provider practices to large hospital primary care and diabetes management settings, facilitating patient-provider communication and understanding.

CHWs are versatile and natural leaders. They can effectively work across community and healthcare providers to accelerate community engagement among underserved populations and structural competency of healthcare providers and, ultimately, lead to patient-centered care and population health improvement for diverse communities.

References

1. Trinh-Shevrin C, Sacks R, Ahn J, Yi SS. Opportunities and challenges in precision medicine: improving cancer prevention and treatment for Asian Americans. J Racial Ethn Health Disparities. 2018;5(1):1–6.
2. Hastings KG, Jose PO, Kapphahn KI, Frank ATH, Goldstein BA, Thompson CA, et al. Leading causes of death among Asian American subgroups (2003–2011). PLoS One [Internet]. 2015;10(4). Available from: https://www.ncbi.nlm.nih.gov/pmc/articles/PMC4411112/
3. King GL, McNeely MJ, Thorpe LE, Mau MLM, Ko J, Liu LL, et al. Understanding and addressing unique needs of diabetes in Asian Americans, native Hawaiians, and Pacific Islanders. Diabetes Care. 2012;35(5):1181–8.
4. Tung EL, Baig AA, Huang ES, Laiteerapong N, Chua K-P. Racial and ethnic disparities in diabetes screening between Asian Americans and other adults: BRFSS 2012–2014. J Gen Intern Med. 2017;32(4):423–9.
5. Islam NS, Kwon SC, Wyatt LC, Ruddock C, Horowitz CR, Devia C, et al. Disparities in diabetes management in Asian Americans in New York City compared with other racial/ethnic minority groups. Am J Public Health. 2015;105(Suppl 3):S443–6.
6. Yi SS, Kwon SC, Sacks R, Trinh-Shevrin C. Commentary: persistence and health-related consequences of the model minority stereotype for Asian Americans. Ethn Dis. 2016;26(1):133–8.
7. Bureau UC. Projections of the size and composition of the U.S: 2014–2060 [Internet]. [cited 2018 Oct 3]. Available from: https://www.census.gov/library/publications/2015/demo/p25-1143.html
8. Bureau USC. American FactFinder – results [Internet]. [cited 2018 Oct 3]. Available from: https://factfinder.census.gov/faces/tableservices/jsf/pages/productview.xhtml?src=bkmk
9. DuBard CA, Gizlice Z. Language spoken and differences in health status, access to care, and receipt of preventive services among US Hispanics. Am J Public Health. 2008;98(11):2021–8.
10. Fiscella K, Franks P, Doescher MP, Saver BG. Disparities in health care by race, ethnicity, and language among the insured: findings from a national sample. Med Care. 2002;40(1):52–9.
11. Kandula NR, Lauderdale DS, Baker DW. Differences in self-reported health among Asians, Latinos, and non-Hispanic whites: the role of language and nativity. Ann Epidemiol. 2007;17(3):191–8.
12. Bureau UC. The Asian Population: 2010 [Internet]. [cited 2018 Oct 3]. Available from: https://www.census.gov/library/publications/2012/dec/c2010br-11.html

13. U.S. Census Bureau. American Fact Finder: 2015 American community survey 1 year estimates, comparative demographic estimates (CP05). 2015; https://factfinder.census.gov.
Accessed 5/1/17, 2017.

14. Mayor's Office of Operations. CEO poverty measure 2005–2014. New York; 2016.

15. Asian American Federation. Profile of New York City's Bangladeshi Americans: 2013 Edition.
2013.

16. Islam N, Riley L, Wyatt L, Tandon SD, Tanner M, Mukherji-Ratnam R, et al. Protocol for the
DREAM Project (Diabetes Research, Education, and Action for Minorities): a randomized
trial of a community health worker intervention to improve diabetic management and control
among Bangladeshi adults in NYC. BMC Public Health. 2014;14:177.

17. Deurenberg P, Deurenberg-Yap M, Guricci S. Asians are different from Caucasians and from
each other in their body mass index/body fat per cent relationship. Obes Rev. 2002;3(3):141–6.

18. Gupta LS, Wu CC, Young S, Perlman SE. Prevalence of diabetes in New York City, 2002–
2008: comparing foreign-born South Asians and other Asians with U.S.-born whites, blacks,
and Hispanics. Diabetes Care. 2011;34(8):1791–3.

19. Yi SS, Kwon SC, Wyatt L, Islam N, Trinh-Shevrin C. Weighing in on the hidden Asian
American obesity epidemic. Prev Med. 2015;73:6–9.

20. NYU Center for the Study of Asian American Health. DREAM Project Materials. https://med.
nyu.edu/asian-health/research/dream/dream-project-materials

21. Islam NS, Tandon D, Mukherji R, Tanner M, Ghosh K, Alam G, et al. Understanding barriers
to and facilitators of diabetes control and prevention in the New York City Bangladeshi community: a mixed-methods approach. Am J Public Health. 2012;102(3):486–90.

22. Trinh-Shevrin C, Kwon SC, Park R, Nadkarni SK, Islam NS. Moving the dial to advance
population health equity in New York City Asian American populations. Am J Public Health.
2015 Jul;105(Suppl 3):e16–25.

23. Islam N, Shapiro E, Wyatt L, Riley L, Zanowiak J, Ursua R, et al. Evaluating community
health workers' attributes, roles, and pathways of action in immigrant communities. Prev Med.
2017;103:1–7.

Part IV

Structural Competency in Policy Advocacy

From Punishment to Public Health: Interdisciplinary Dialogues and Cross-Sector Policy Innovations

Jeffrey Coots, Gary Belkin, and Ernest Drucker

Dismantling the Prison Industrial Complex with the Masters Tools

Early in my law school experience, I realized it wasn't enough. Despite the Constitution's promise of equal protection and the legislative gains of the civil rights movement, I came to understand that the practice of law remained primarily a tool of economic suppression and racial oppression. No matter how good a defense attorney I became, the deck would always be stacked against my clients. The mandatory minimum sentences, the prosecutorial discretion to plea bargain, a power structure so dependent on racism it seemed to drip from the walls of the courtroom and reverberate from the bars of the prison cell—we didn't stand a chance. How could my colleagues and I pull people away from a system designed so well to keep them coming back, again and again?

Thankfully, my law school offered a joint degree program with a local medical school, and about a dozen of my classmates and I broadened our disciplinary reach to include a public health framework. We grappled with population health

J. Coots (✉)
Department of Criminal Justice, John Jay College of Criminal Justice, City University of New York, New York City, NY, USA
e-mail: jcoots@jjay.cuny.edu

G. Belkin
NYC Department of Health and Mental Hygiene, New York City, NY, USA

Department of Psychiatry, New York University School of Medicine, New York City, NY, USA

E. Drucker
New York University, College of Global Public Health, New York City, NY, USA

Montefiore Medical Center / Albert Einstein College of Medicine, New York City, NY, USA

© Springer Nature Switzerland AG 2019
H. Hansen, J. M. Metzl (eds.), *Structural Competency in Mental Health and Medicine*,
https://doi.org/10.1007/978-3-030-10525-9_15

approaches alongside nurses, dentists, occupational and physical therapists, physicians, and social workers. I learned to confront policy and practice misalignments instead of episodic behavioral provocations, and I was exposed to a social determinants framework that directed my gaze further upstream than street-based police encounters and courtroom deal-making. Several of the public health advocates I met were even beginning to pay more attention to the epidemic that brought me to law school in the first place. By the time I graduated, the phenomenon commonly known as "mass incarceration" was recognized as a public health problem of disastrous proportions—and one largely borne by poor and minority communities [1, 2].

I arrived in New York City in 2013 to find scores of committed, knowledgeable, and creative practitioners, academics, and researchers who recognized the dangers of overcriminalizing urban environments and populations. Despite this knowledge, the allies I encountered working in medicine, law, public health, and criminal justice often struggled to achieve the policy reforms they viewed as vital to the health and wellness of their clients and communities. The "punishment paradigm" was seemingly intractable. Two of the first people I met held distinct ideas about how to change this paradigm.

Bridging Siloes and Accelerating Innovation

Dr. Ernest Drucker learned to engage the criminal justice system out of necessity. He founded Montefiore Hospital's 1000-patient drug treatment program in 1970 and served as its director until 1990. During that time, most of his patients were arrested, incarcerated, and eventually released back into his care. Too often, they returned to him sicker than when they left. From 1980 to 2005, Dr. Drucker served as the Director of the Division of Public Health and Policy Research at Montefiore/Einstein. In this role he documented the increased physical and mental health challenges facing incarcerated populations and contributed to a growing body of evidence indicating that these challenges are often worsened by prolonged justice system involvement with its attendant interruptions of health care, family and social supports, and multiple traumatic events, including continued exposure to violence while in custody.

Dr. Drucker's idea on how to change the incarceration paradigm was to share this knowledge in multidisciplinary settings and charge systems actors with articulating sensible policy and practice reforms to alleviate the suffering of those involved. He recognized that the siloed nature of health delivery systems, criminal justice agencies, public health apparatuses, and academic institutions prevented meaningful collaboration to improve outcomes for individuals that cut across all these sectors. If we were to build bridges across these siloes, we needed to start by learning how to talk to each other, how to unpack existing policy structures we understood to be creating harm, and how to collaborate in meaningful ways to reform not just one system but many intersecting systems. So I began working with Dr. Drucker to construct a "classroom without walls" where these learnings could begin to take shape. We called it *The Academy of Public Health and Criminal Justice*.

When I first met Dr. Gary Belkin, he was the Behavioral Health Medical Director of NYC Health + Hospitals, which is the City's largest provider of mental health and drug treatment services through its 11 hospitlas and numerous outpatient programs, and includes responsibility to those who were too sick to be treated in the local jail system while awaiting trial. Dr. Belkin was also an Associate Professor in Psychiatry at New York University School of Medicine, where he led the program on Global Mental Health, which was designed to advance innovative implementation and policy approaches to scale and improve population mental health strategies. In both roles, he lead efforts to extend the impacts of behavioral health sciences on other social sectors and outcomes, including homelessness, street-level gun violence, and early childhood.

Dr. Belkin's idea on how to change the incarceration paradigm was that we already knew what needed to change, but we were still too poorly equipped and unimaginative to do it. He argued that we actually know a lot about how a range of social determinants of health become key factors in social pathology, criminal behaviors, and imprisonment and some of what works to intervene and act on those connections. But we lack the operational and political capacities to routinely use and scale what works and ambitiously move resources from a punishment to a public health paradigm. Dr. Belkin introduced me to a suite of quality improvement tools that could help accelerate innovation at the intersections of public health and criminal justice, and we began looking for partners for our first test case in New York City.

Pushing the Paradigm: From Punishment to Public Health

In 2013, with the help and guidance of Dr. Belkin and Dr. Drucker, and with crucial leadership from Jeremy Travis, an international expert on prisoner reentry, we launched a paradigm-shifting collaborative initiative under the umbrella theme *From Punishment to Public Health*, or P2PH. This group of academic, research, policy, and direct service agencies joined together in 2013 to address the myriad public health and safety challenges flowing from the overuse of incarceration as a means of social control. We worked to develop a mutual focus on the endemic social and structural problems that lead to incarceration and to reimagine the features of institutions and policymaking that position public health interventions to be held accountable to better health, safety, and social outcomes and to reduce the risk of criminal and antisocial behaviors. In utilizing a two-pronged approach of interdisciplinary dialogues and practice innovation accelerators, P2PH's platform offers examples of how to engage medical students and faculty in local advocacy opportunities that reach outside the four walls of clinical practice.

In working to integrate policy and practice across these sectors, P2PH members regularly confront four key challenges resulting from the silo effect described above. The first, most obvious challenge is one of language practitioners use different words and phrases to describe the same behaviors and/or clients. The second key obstacle arises from the different training and skills of the practitioners in each sector, as shaped through their formal education and on-the-job training and cultural assimilation. Of course, the "skills gap" between disciplines reinforces the "language gap" across sectors, and these two challenges are best addressed in tandem.

For example, one of the first issues addressed by P2PH was the high rates of arrest among homeless individuals seeking shelter in New York City's sprawling subway system. Two main sets of actors are responsible for addressing this issue in the field: homeless outreach workers and police officers. Outreach workers are drawn primarily from social work backgrounds and are trained to assess clients by first looking at their feet to identify signs of bodily distress—swelling, discoloration, scaling, etc. They speak in clinical terms about the safety of a given individual vis-à-vis their surroundings and current psychological state. In contrast, police officers tend to study law enforcement as undergraduates and are trained in the Police Academy to assess potential for danger by looking at a person's hands. They communicate with each other about the danger one such person might present to others in the subway. In beginning to work on this issue, it was vital for P2PH members to understand the gaps in language and skills between these two groups and strive to close those gaps in order to engender trust and collaboration among the key stakeholders. P2PH's work on this project is described in more detail below in *Cross-Sector Policy Innovations*.

The third major challenge in overcoming the silo effect is the differing responses to common problems that have become the "standard operating procedure" in respective disciplines (e.g., psychopathology vs. crime, treat vs. arrest), and the fourth key challenge is the stark difference in metrics of success defined by practitioners and policymakers in each sector. These challenges are also linked and must be addressed on parallel tracks, since defining success necessarily shapes activities in pursuit thereof. Keeping with the subway analogy above, outreach workers attempt to engage clients in a conversation about their wants and needs with the goal of convincing the client to accept a placement into a short-term housing facility with attendant social service supports. The workers track their "touches" with clients and the number of placements they facilitate each night and are ultimately responsible for facilitating pathways to housing services on a voluntary basis for individuals who are considered "chronically" homeless. In contrast, police officers will remind individuals they are not allowed to engage in certain types of behaviors (e.g., lying down, panhandling, etc.) in the transit system and can offer transportation to the main intake shelter or call an ambulance for someone in severe need of medical attention. Officers track arrests, service offers, and acceptances and assist with medical emergencies. They are ultimately responsible for ensuring public safety within the subway system, a metric of success much broader than can be fully achieved through better solutions for homelessness. This disparity of scope in metrics of success is a key learning of the P2PH initiative itself—we, as a society, are simply asking police officers to do too much, and we all share culpability when they fall short.

If we are to fully integrate public health and public safety aims, diverse groups of stakeholders will need to embrace new responsibilities and new measures of accountability. As outlined below, this process begins with interdisciplinary dialogues that allow actors across sectors to develop a common language and framework for shared problems, followed by cross-trainings to promote shared skills and competencies. Only then can we begin to develop collaborative responses that allow us to be held accountable to a common set of metrics that define our shared success.

Interdisciplinary Dialogues

Invigorated by our early attempts at building bridges across disciplines and expertise, Dr. Drucker and several members of the P2PH team set out to replicate these interdisciplinary conversations. Throughout the remainder of 2013 and 2014, under the umbrella of the Academy of Public Health and Criminal Justice, we hosted more than a dozen gatherings of interdisciplinary faculty, students, and practitioners. Attendees set out to identify opportunities for collaborative research projects that push the traditional boundaries of criminal justice and public health discourse, leading to the organic formation of several new projects examining issues such as the inclusion of criminal justice involvement in community health assessments, the impact of various carceral settings on inmate competency evaluations, and the secondary psychological effects on health workers serving inmates subjected to solitary confinement.

At the outset of this series, presentations and discussions were based on the existing NYC issues and programs that affected all—enabling health professionals and academics to better understand law enforcement and criminal justice perspectives. As the events progressed to wider audiences of stakeholders and presenters, P2PH welcomed practitioners and scholars from across North America and Europe to demonstrate their attempts at resolving similar issues. Our first large-scale conference, in 2014, proposed a reframing of "prisoner reentry" through a public health and epidemiological lens of "decarceration." Several members of NYC's academic and practice communities contributed to a full-day discussion focused on bridging the divide between health and justice sectors. Panelists recognized that while many good collaborations were already in existence, community-based capacity continued to be far outstripped by demand for affordable housing, stable employment, educational opportunities, and competent physical and behavioral health services. Shortfalls in these systems and sectors were recognized as the main drivers of criminal and antisocial behaviors in poor and mostly minority neighborhoods in the city.

P2PH's second major conference event was hosted at Brooklyn Borough Hall in 2015, with welcome remarks from Borough President Eric Adams, a strong advocate and policymaker focused on community health and criminal justice issues. Dr. Belkin, co-chair of the P2PH Steering Committee, spearheaded this event to highlight transformative governance strategies in public mental health and invited several of his international colleagues to present their successes in leveraging government resources to impact cross-sector mental health challenges. In creating a dynamic event, Dr. Belkin, who had since left Health + Hospitals to be the Executive Deputy Commissioner at the New York City Department of Health and Mental Hygiene, was instrumental in engaging First Lady Chirlane McCray, who utilized the Keynote Presentation as a platform to call for a "road map" to a more inclusive mental health system. This effort evolved into ThriveNYC, which invested an estimated $850M in its first four years to stimulate a broader public health approach to mental health, with an array of 54 initiatives that range from parenting to police, e.g. scaled promotion of early child socio-emotional learning, building capacity for health responses rather than polic responses to behavioral health emergencies. ThriveNYC consists of several platforms including training in Mental Health First Aid, investing more in early childhood interventions, closing treatment gaps in poor communities, partnering with community organizations to drive reforms, using data in better ways to track improvements and persistent gaps, and strengthening governments' ability to lead and engage broader networks of communities for change. It also established the NYC Mental Health Council comprised of almost two dozen agencies to better address mental health at structural and cross-sector levels, and treat it like the intersectional issue that it is.

P2PH's Third Annual Conference, in 2016, was delivered in partnership with the Behavioral Health Diversion Forum, a group that meets quarterly to coordinate efforts between court-based law enforcement personnel and community-based behavioral health service providers. While the first two conference events focused mainly on developing a shared language and vision of integrated policy and practice, the third conference had explicit workforce training goals aimed at growing the community-based capacity to meet the needs of justice-involved clients with behavioral health challenges. Day one of the event drew over 200 managerial and frontline staff members from over 60 NYC agencies to participate in 9 panel sessions that included 6 medical clinicians (MDs) and 5 city/state policymakers. Day two's focus on "Systems Integration Planning" welcomed local and state policymakers, clinical directors, and community partners to participate in creative discussions aimed at increasing and accelerating linkages across systems of care (including those within carceral settings). The well-balanced breadth and depth of the event lead to agreement among the partners to deliver a similar, more sophisticated event in 2017, and efforts to organize a series of learning communities to allow for more regular learning and cross-sector dialogues among these key agencies and their respective workforces.

Feedback from P2PH conference participants consistently notes the unique cross-sector nature of presentations and other attendees. The events are recognized as excellent networking opportunities for those trying to exert influence outside of their own field or develop their own interdisciplinary practice and perspective. Perhaps most importantly, by fostering dialogue and learning across sectors and disciplines, these events address the first two main challenges to cross-sector collaboration—shared language and skills—and lay the groundwork for more direct policy and practice innovations such as those described below.

Cross-Sector Policy Innovations

As noted above, several medical school faculty members now sit on the P2PH Steering Committee, and they regularly participate in efforts to integrate practice across sectors. Dr. Belkin co-chaired the committee along with Jeremy Travis, then President of John Jay College of Criminal Justice. Dr. Belkin and President Travis were instrumental in stimulating agency-level policy changes that led to the creation of a pre-arrest diversion program focused on homeless individuals seeking shelter in New York City's subway systems and opening the door for P2PH to pursue similar policy innovation projects in the future.

Early in the de Blasio Administration, President Travis reached out to newly appointed Police Commissioner William Bratton and introduced the P2PH consortium along with our desire to facilitate a pre-arrest diversion program in NYC. Commissioner Bratton responded warmly and assigned the Deputy Commissioner of Collaborative Policing, Susan Herman, to participate in the new P2PH Diversion working group. Other members of the group included the NYC Department of Health and Mental Hygiene, the New York University Langone Medical Center, the New York County District Attorney's Office, the New York Academy of Medicine, and the Vera Institute of Justice. The initial charge to the group was simple: identify subpopulations of individuals at risk for arrest that could safely and effectively be diverted from arrest toward some type of public health or social support service offering. Rather quickly, members of the group identified the transit system, particularly the subway system, as an opportunity ripe for innovation, especially in terms of responding to homeless individuals seeking shelter and facing arrest for relatively minor offenses.

Group membership then expanded to include additional agencies with direct control of the transit environment and content expertise in working with homeless populations, including NYC Department of Homeless Services (DHS), the NYC Transit Authority, the Metropolitan Transportation Authority, and Bowery Residents' Committee (BRC). Single adults in New York City have "right to shelter" based on a 1981 court settlement and DHS contracts with local nonprofits, such as BRC, to facilitate placements for those in need. The working group analyzed arrest patterns and resulting court dispositions, police officer survey and focus group findings, train system delays, and existing homeless outreach resources before scanning national best practices in pre-arrest diversion practices and protocols.

Throughout these efforts, the group developed a common lexicon to articulate the shared challenge of homeless individuals seeking shelter in the subway system and analyzed the skills of those involved in existing response efforts—police officers and homeless outreach workers. Robust engagement with NYPD's managerial and frontline transit officers throughout the design and launch of this project served to further strengthen the working relationships between BRC, NYC Transit, and NYPD, and regular cross-trainings of NYPD officers and BRC outreach workers bolstered fidelity to the joint patrol model designed by the working group. In preparation for the busier winter season, BRC facilitated 10 trainings to more than 200 officers in late 2015 and early 2016 and repeated these cross-training efforts in fall, 2016.

In developing a coordinated response and a common set of metrics to define success, P2PH introduced a set of quality improvement strategies familiar to most health service personnel. Dr. Belkin's persistent focus on the small-step redesign process enabled P2PH to advocate for accelerated policy and practice changes to the coordination between New York City Police Department officers and homeless outreach workers at BRC. The group designed and tested a joint patrol design involving two police officers and two BRC outreach workers canvassing train cars and subway platforms for vulnerable citizens. As a result, homeless individuals sleeping overnight on the subway, particularly those with potential psychiatric symptoms, are now directed by a joint patrol team of police and outreach workers to respite beds, transitional housing facilities, and mental health assessment units rather than arrest.

Recognizing the strength of this collaborative model, NYPD designated officers in each of its transit districts to serve as liaisons to homeless service providers and participate in these types of joint patrols. This initiative, which has placed over 1200 clients since its launch in fall 2014, is jointly funded by DHS, MTA, and DOHMH. It serves as a model for the ways that medical school faculty and public health administrators can collaborate with non-health sectors to make meaningful, health-promoting changes in institutional procedures.

The Fundamentals of Cross-Systems Learning and Innovation

P2PH members and partners have elicited several key learnings over 4 years of interdisciplinary dialogues and cross-sector policy innovations. As mentioned above, our pre-arrest diversion work has laid bare the fact that we have unfairly (and unwisely) piled on a plethora of roles and responsibilities for law enforcement to handle, and we all bear some of the blame for phenomena like mass incarceration and over-policing of black and brown neighborhoods. Those of us not familiar with working closely with law enforcement were pleasantly surprised by the focus group and survey findings that officers not only wanted to build their own skills in confronting difficult social situations not well resolved with arrest and sanction but that they overwhelmingly welcomed other practitioners to stand by their side while doing so. This bodes well for future efforts seeking to reduce the criminalization of poverty, substance misuse, mental illness, and other structurally related phenomena.

The process of interdisciplinary dialogues and skills sharing also serves to build trust among practitioners, researchers, and policymakers that may not have a strong history of cooperation. Simply talking through differences of opinion and discovering new terminology for familiar phenomena can serve as a powerful tool in breaking down silos and identifying common ground on which to build. Engendering this trust goes a long way to constructing a shared framework around a given problem and developing a set of common aims that guide the creation of new collaborative responses and related metrics of success.

Application to Other Situations

The key challenges discussed in the context of P2PH's work to overcome silos in municipal governance structure—language, skills, responses, and metrics—overlay nicely with the five core structural competencies discussed by Drs. Metzl and Hansen in "Structural Competency: Theorizing a new medical engagement with stigma and inequality" (2014). The ability to recognize structural forces that impact health coupled with a fluency in non-clinical language to articulate these structures are necessary preconditions to participating in cross-sector initiatives such as P2PH. The medical school faculty counted among the P2PH Steering Committee members brought these tools with them to our first meetings.

At the early meetings of the pre-arrest diversion working group, several members identified the homeless clients as "hard to serve" or "service-resistant" individuals. Other members, particularly those with greater ability to articulate cultural presentations in structural terms, pushed back on this framing and suggested instead that the services currently offered were not appropriate for engaging this particular subset of clients. This reframing helped us to discuss the standard responses in a different light, with a focus on the different types of responses and resources we could offer clients rather than a tactical discussion about how to overcome a perceived "hardened resistance." This in turn opened the way for the group to imagine structural interventions that aligned with this framing of the issue. In the end, we identified several types of short-term shelter options that were preferable to the large intake shelter that was the default offering.

Finally, on the issue of humility, P2PH's position within the City University of New York offers several distinct advantages. Whereas clinicians and policymakers are expected to provide concrete answers and solutions to the immediate problems presented by their clients and constituents, liberal arts academic settings allow for nuanced discourse of policy-level issues, in which the inquiry itself is often valued above the resulting recommendations. Indeed, P2PH has come to be known as a neutral convener of cross-systems stakeholders facing complex challenges that defy simple solutions. By offering a safe space to voice realpolitik operational impediments to improved outcomes, P2PH engages practitioners in unique ways that can generate hope and excitement in the face of seemingly daunting obstacles. Among our members, there is a growing recognition that together we can overcome our siloed natures and develop meaningful, durable solutions to the most pressing challenges of the day.

References

1. Warren, J., et al. One in 100: Behind Bars in America 2008. Washington, DC: The Pew Center on the States; 2018.
2. Drucker E. A plague of prisons: the epidemiology of mass incarceration in America. Reprint edition. New York: The New Press; 2013.

Agents of Change: How Allied Healthcare Workers Transform Inequalities in the Healthcare Industry

Alethia Jones

The Problem

Poverty pay in hospitals

In 2014, 2000 service and maintenance workers at Johns Hopkins Medical Center halted work for 3 days during contract negotiations. 1199SEIU called the strike to highlight "poverty wages" that forced full-time employees to obtain public assistance to make ends meet.

In These Times quoted Dr. Benjamin Oldfield, a resident who led doctors, medical and nursing students in supporting the striking workers: "[W]e know that financial insecurity leads to bad health outcomes. For a place like Hopkins, which has plenty of money, I'm surprised that they haven't gotten this one right yet" [1].

Source: "Striking Workers Shame Prestigious Johns Hopkins Hospital Over Low Pay." *In These Times*. April 10, 2014.

Healthcare institutions mirror society's inequalities. At almost one-fifth of the US economy [2], health industry employers generate the very inequalities that clinicians then "treat" as individual cases of illness. As a society, we value caring rhetorically but have formal structures and robust belief systems that devalue those who do care work [3]. Allied health workers have played a critical role in compelling the industry to address the structural inequalities in its own backyard. They fought workplace norms, industry rationales, and federal laws that reinforced their place at the bottom rung of the healthcare hierarchy. They transformed low-wage, dead-end jobs into living wage career ladders. Today, they are on the front lines of new

A. Jones (✉)
Open Society Foundations Fellowships Program, New York, NY, USA

© Springer Nature Switzerland AG 2019
H. Hansen, J. M. Metzl (eds.), *Structural Competency in Mental Health and Medicine*,
https://doi.org/10.1007/978-3-030-10525-9_16

models of care that strengthen innovative efforts in community health. This case invites clinicians to see their workplaces as sites of deep structural inequality with significant impact on workers, communities, and patient health.

Theoretical Framework

How can we end the healthcare sector's role as a central generator of structural inequalities? Allied health workers are "agents of change" who have disrupted the status quo and secured structural redistribution of resources in the industry. Breakthrough changes occurred in the 1960s when they partnered with the southern civil rights movement to bring an end to their second-class status. The industry will expand robustly in the coming decades, but most healthcare jobs remain low-wage and not unionized [4]. By sharing this history and contemporary examples, practitioners can gain insights into forging structural partnerships that match the size and scale of inequality within the industry's midst. Clinicians, along with trustees and administrators, can either transform structural barriers in the industry or perpetuate the subordinate status of many workers. The case concludes with four principles for forging effective partnerships with allied health workers.

This case incorporates the voices of the allied workforce to furnish a "bottom-up" view of their struggles to transform exploitative healthcare jobs into sustainable employment. No one is more acutely aware of the precarity experienced by these workers than the workers themselves. It uses historical and contemporary accounts of union organizing by healthcare workers in New York City and at Johns Hopkins Hospital in Baltimore to illustrate challenges to making structural changes in the industry.

The Path

Unionization is the primary vehicle to alter the structure of opportunity for low-wage healthcare workers. The allied health workforce includes all service, maintenance, and clerical positions as well as paraprofessional and professional titles, such as nurses, social workers, lab technicians, and pharmacists.[1] They are overwhelmingly female, immigrant, and people of color. 1199SEIU is the largest healthcare workers union local in the USA. Founded in 1932 as Local 1199 in New York City, this union of pharmacy workers branched into hospital worker organizing in the 1950s. The union's history captures core features of worker experiences because of the union's presence in New York City's major hospitals; its experience as a national union organizing all across the country; and its presence in nursing homes, home care agencies, laboratories, pharmacies, clinics, as well as hospitals. In 2017, it had 400,000 members in hospitals (including academic medical centers), nursing homes, home care agencies, clinics, and community health centers in five states (FL, MA, MD, NJ, NY) and Washington, DC. The Service Employees International

---

[1] Definitions vary but often include sub-baccalaureate positions and jobs regarded as semi- and unskilled.

Union (SEIU) represents one million healthcare workers nationwide, including the Committee of Interns and Residents and the Doctors Council.[2]

Challenge: Healthcare Work as Low-Wage Work

Today's healthcare personnel infrastructure reflects assumptions rooted in the industry's origins in charity care and noblesse oblige. Hospitals originated in the seventeenth century in India, the Middle East, and Europe from the philanthropic impulses of monarchs, the wealthy, and religious orders. As such, they served the very poor, the disabled, the elderly, the insane, the socially isolated, and soldiers. For everyone else, healthcare occurred at home with visits from local doctors when needed. In the USA, the landed gentry (like Benjamin Franklin) and religious institutions created hospitals out of a charitable impulse to serve the less fortunate. At a later period, the connection to charity and voluntarism was further cemented when the nation's poorhouses were converted to hospitals, nursing homes, and state mental institutions. For example, New York City's famed Bellevue Hospital began as the Almshouse Hospital in 1736 [5–7].

From the outset, working in hospitals was as an act of charity. While hospitals' reliance on donations from wealthy benefactors is well-known, the compulsory "donations" of the poor to the financial viability of healthcare institutions is largely invisible. Initially, nuns and lay volunteers (often unmarried women) volunteered to feed, clean, and tend to the ill and dying. They were soon joined by impoverished former patients who stayed on after they recuperated in exchange for room and board. In addition, inmates of poorhouses were assigned to work at hospitals to earn their stay (similar to prison work release programs) [8, 9].[3] As a result, the earliest hospital "workers" were literally charity cases.

These workers' simultaneous reliance on public assistance while working at the hospital was a widely accepted norm. As hospitals grew in size, wealth, and status, nuns and lay volunteers cobbled together an informal personnel apparatus rooted in charitable paternalism to manage their growing workforce. Workers lived in hospital dormitories and basements with little privacy or time off.[4] Tasks, hours, hiring, and firing were meted out in an arbitrary blend of benevolence and reprimand, all at impossibly low wages [10, 11]. Neither workers, managers, nor trustees imagined a living wage as appropriate.

Most significantly, federal and state laws institutionalized the indentured servitude of hospital workers. In the 1930s, the American Hospital Association

---

[2] There are also unions for nurses and for workers in public hospitals and healthcare centers. To learn more about SEIU affiliated healthcare unions, visit www.1199seiu.org, www.seiu.org as well as www.doctorscouncil.org and www.cirseiu.org.

[3] Prior to federal New Deal and Great Society social assistance programs, local taxes funded poorhouses that warehoused the orphaned, the homeless, the disabled, and the elderly. Residents were forced to work at nearby establishments (like rock quarries) to generate revenue as taxpayer dollars did not cover all their operating costs (see Eubanks 2018 for a brief history).

[4] For example, as part of its expansion in 1913, Mount Sinai authorized the construction of a dorm for 240 of its employees, including nurses (Hirsh and Doherty 1952).

successfully lobbied Congress to exempt nonprofit hospital workers from minimum wage laws, social security benefits, and the right to unionize [12]. In the South, hospitals were segregated. In the North, the mass migrations of African American sharecroppers from the South and immigrants from the Caribbean, Latin America, and Asia provided a new influx of poor workers who replaced the "charity cases" of a previous era.

Hospitals benefited significantly from the post-World War II economic boom. Scientific discoveries fueled their growth. In addition, they gained new revenue from private health insurance, publicly funded health programs (Medicaid, Medicare, veterans health), government research grants, and the generosity of corporate titans. Services to an expanding middle class and to wealthy patrons seeking cutting edge treatments replaced their historic emphasis on serving the poor.

The unquestioned reliance on an impoverished, charity-dependent workforce quietly subsidized the rise of the modern healthcare industry. To oversee their rapidly growing workforce, hospital leaders recruited hotel managers to join their management teams. Hospitals and hotels shared a "plantation ideal" model of services where patrons recuperated in comfort while tended to by a bevy of cooks and maids [13] (Fig. 1).

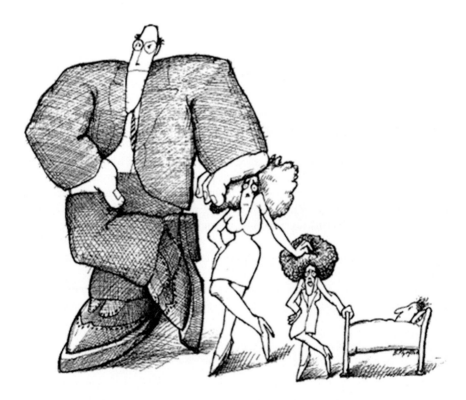

Fig. 1 The healthcare hierarchy. (Source: Illustration by Bill Plympton for Health Policy Advisory Center. Circa 1970 in *Health/PAC Bulletin*. Access at http://www.healthpacbulletin.org/plymptoons/. Credit ©The Health/PAC Digital Archive. Permission pending)

In this social and historical milieu, the paternalism of charity care easily married with the social practices of Jim Crow. A Department of Labor study of hospital wages in 16 metropolitan areas in 1956–1957 found low salaries as the norm, with New York City paying an average of 84 cents an hour with female workers in similar jobs earning even less [12]. Only five locations in the USA paid over $1.00 an hour. Journalist A.H. Raskin noted that, "…it was a tragic joke in the hospitals that none of their nonprofessional employees could afford to be sick" [14] (Fig. 2). An industry assessment concluded:

> Hospitals have long been the urban employer of last resort. The newcomers, the discriminated-against, those who are excluded from other jobs are likely to end up as porters, nurses' aides, orderlies, kitchen help, housekeepers, and the like, in the immense and rapidly growing hospital industry. … Hours are long, duties dirty and boring, job security non-existent. …[T]urnover rates often approach 90 percent per year. [15]

By the 1950s and 1960s, the gendered and racial pay gaps reflected the firm hierarchy of race, gender, and class that structured the system. Pay gaps institutionalized "common sense" beliefs that perceive care work (including child care, teaching, and domestic work) as natural extensions of women's roles as mothers and classified it as "unskilled" or semiskilled labor. This web of laws, social practices, and popular beliefs reinforced the assumption that these workers should be grateful to work under any condition without complaint.

It is well knowm that the hospital worker hierarchy features well paid, highly trained, white men at the top; intermediate paid, largely white, women in the middle: and poorly paid, black and brown women at the bottom. The following chart gives the details.

Job	% of total Employment (1)	% of total payroll (1)	pay range ($ per week) (2)	approximate % female (3)	approximate % non-white (4)
management/supervisory	9	13	200-500	15-20	10-20
academic	2	5	200-400	20	5
interns/residents	6	9	180-250	10	8
staff RN's	21	25	155-170	98	40
Lab techs	10	9	135-165	75	40
LPN's	7	7	110-130	85	90
clerical	11	8	100-130	85	60
aides/manual service	34	24	95-115	80	80

Notes: (1) figures refer to New York University Hospital; (2) figures are for New York City short-term, non-governmental hospitals, spring 1970; (3) figures are for U.S.; (4) figures are for New York City Municipal hospitals.

Fig. 2 Gender and race hierarchies reflected in hospital pay scales. (Source: Data compiled by Health Policy Advisory Center researchers. In "Hospital Unions: A Long Time Coming." *Health/PAC Bulletin*. July–August 1970. See www.healthpacbulletin.org. Credit ©The Health/PAC Digital Archive. Permission pending)

These structures persist. In 2014, as 1199SEIU negotiated a contract with Johns Hopkins Hospital, workers shared their stories of living in homeless shelters or doubled up with relatives. Others faced eviction and received food stamps and other forms of public assistance to make ends meet (see www.hardshipathopkins.org). Today's home care industry also reflects a marriage of work and welfare. Initiated in the 1970s as an innovative welfare to work experiment, the federal government's new home care program required welfare recipients to care for poverty stricken, homebound elderly and disabled patients [16, 17]. Consequently, the low wages of this female workforce produced significant savings while addressing a growing healthcare need. Today, many home care workers are disproportionately women of color, immigrant and undocumented. Those with legal status often earn minimum wage and rely on public assistance (such as public housing and food stamps) to make ends meet.

Response: Unionization Because Workers' Lives Matter

Durable structural inequality at Johns Hopkins 1969 and 2014

Annie Henry, an instrument processor, remembers when she and her co-workers at Johns Hopkins voted to unionize in 1969. Only on staff for 6 months, she recalls, "I was ready to quit. The hospital was like a plantation. You couldn't even talk to supervisors." She and other workers were heartened when the recently widowed Coretta Scott King stood with them during the 1969 strike which linked the fight for civil rights with worker rights.

Annie also participated in the 2014 strike at Johns Hopkins and lamented: "Never in forty-five years did I think I'd still be doing this. We want to be paid our worth."

Sources: "50 Who Carried the 1199 Torch: Profiles of our Pioneers," *Our Life and Times: A Journal of 1199SEIU,* December 2009 and "Baltimore Since Beth Steel: Hopkins Hospital Workers Fight for 15," *Dissent,* June 26, 2014.

By the 1950s, healthcare workers were treated as disposable workers with jobs characterized by high turnover and total subservience. Workers found the ability to question the status quo and the courage to confront this oppressive system in collective action. In 1958, after decades of winning victories for pharmacy workers, Local 1199's membership voted to focus on the hospital sector to end the exploitation there. The union's organizing staff spent a decade cajoling and persuading hospital workers to believe in their own worth. Hospital workers drew direct inspiration and support from the civil rights movement in the South. Dubbed "Soul Power," the union combined classic tactics of worker organizing with the rhetoric and strategies of civil rights activism [13]. They began to see their situations in structural rather than individual terms, rejecting the ideology of individual efforts as *the* path to success (Fig. 3).

In 1968, 1199 members won the nation's first ever hospital worker contract. It tripled wages (to a minimum of $100 a week) and provided healthcare, pension, and education benefits to 40,000 members at multiple New York City hospitals.

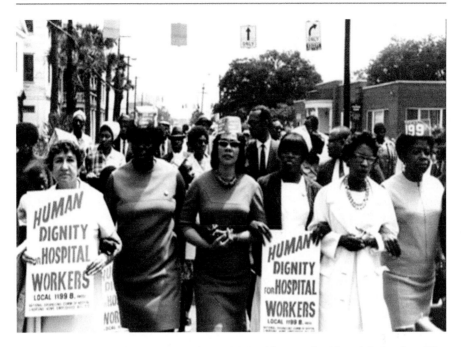

Fig. 3 "Soul Power" – Civil rights and workers' rights. *The recently widowed Coretta Scott King (center) marches with hospital workers in Charleston, South Carolina during their 1969 strike. She is joined by Mary Moultrie, a nurse's aide and president of South Carolina 1199B (second from the left) and Doris Turner, president of Local 1199 (first on the right).* (Source: 1199 photo archives. Credit: © Jim Tynan. Reprinted with permission)

Professional titles joined the union because as Ann Flack, a registered nurse noted: "...nurses wanted what the unionized maintenance staff had" – paid sick days, regular time off, benefits, and a voice in improving patient care [18].

1199 launched a national campaign to unionize hospital workers across the nation. By 1985, 150,000 members in 20 states joined the union. The turn to unions meant workers no longer relied on the kindness and charity of individual supervisors in their efforts to get a fair deal. The power of their collective voices proved to be the only the vehicle to obtain concrete and lasting results.

Challenge: Employers Defend the Status Quo

Healthcare leaders' paternalism seek to preserve and protect the status quo
"This is not a strike, but a revolution against law and order."
 Greater New York Hospital Association, 1959
 Source: "1852–2002: The Sesquicentennial," Mount Sinai Hospital 150th Anniversary Committee (2002: 23).

Employers vigorously defended existing norms when confronted with worker demands instead of interrogating the assumptions of the socioeconomic system they inherited. In 1958, every nonprofit hospital in New York City (except one) refused to allow their workers to vote on unionization. In a 1959 letter, Mount Sinai's leadership explained: "A hospital is not an economic, industrial unit. It is a social unit. … Human life should not be a pawn in jousting for economic gain or power." Hospital executives asked, "…strike against whom—our patients, sick people, children needing immediate medical care!" [19]. In 2014, Johns Hopkins's president, Ronald Peterson, conveyed the sentiments of a benevolent employer who saw current arrangements as essentially fair, even exemplary. In an op-ed in *The Baltimore Sun*, he insisted that each employee is "…part of our team and vital to the world-class care we provide." He lauded existing wages for service and maintenance workers for being above the federal ($7.50) and state ($10.10) minimum wages. He drew attention to health benefits and educational programs that give unskilled, low-wage workers and their families opportunities for self-improvement [20]. Others suggested that the requested $15 minimum wage would cost Hopkins $3 million annually, a small fraction of its reported $145 million surplus [1, 21].

Response: Strikes Compel Change from Charity to Justice

Strikes and civil disobedience – violating existing laws to get justice – yield results

From the *New York Times* obituary on Leon Davis:

…[He] was more than a founder and president of Local 1199 of the Drug, Hospital and Health Care Employees Union: he was a virtual patriarch to its generations of clerks, janitors, aides, orderlies, laundry workers, porters, dishwashers, elevator operators and other low profile employees in hospitals, nursing homes and pharmacies. In a turbulent half-century at the helm, he led major walkouts in New York in 1959 and 1962 and in Charleston, S.C., in 1969, was twice jailed for defying anti-strike injunctions, helped overturn Federal and state laws that exempted health care workers from collective bargaining, and was instrumental in raising the wages, working conditions, living standards and dignity of thousands he called America's forgotten workers [22].

Source: "Leon Davis, 85, Head of Health-Care Union, Dies." *The New York Times*. September 15, 1992.

Workers faced an enormous power imbalance economically, socially, and ideologically. They were excluded from all labor protections and it was illegal for them to strike. To end their invisibility, pierce the veil of complacency, and get their side of the story out to the public, workers went on strike. Because reasoned arguments failed, strikes proved the only effective vehicle to gain public attention to the immorality of accepted norms.

Six months after virtually every hospital refused to allow workers to vote for a union, 3500 workers from seven New York City nonprofit hospitals went on strike for 46 days. Employers created a committee to discuss their demands. After 3 years of dialogue, no changes in working conditions resulted. A second city-wide, multi-employer strike occurred in 1962 and lasted 56 days. The 113-day strike in Charleston, South Carolina, in 1969 resulted in 1000 arrests, hunger strikes in jail, and national television coverage [13].

The need to strike persists. In 2014, Johns Hopkins endured months of negative mainstream and social media attention to its poverty wages, including a 3-day strike and a high-profile Mothers' Day March and Rally that featured worker testimonies and support from celebrities like Danny Glover. To avert a second 3-day strike, Maryland's governor intervened and forced the parties to the negotiating table where they successfully settled. Union members with 20 years or more of experience received an immediate $15-an-hour minimum wage. Others would make at least $13 an hour by 2018, well above the $12.25 minimum Hopkins offered [23].

> **Health care workers continue to rely on public assistance to survive**
> Kiva Robbins, an environmental services worker at Johns Hopkins Hospital, in her letter to the editor of *The Baltimore Sun* asked: "Is it fair that workers who spend their entire careers in dietary or housekeeping jobs must live in poverty?" She wondered why her salary was only $12.20 an hour after 12 years of service. She had taken advantage of educational opportunities and earned a certificate, but she could not afford the child care she needed to take additional college classes to earn a degree. Moreover, she found Johns Hopkins's fabulous healthcare benefits "beyond my means" and instead relied on "Maryland taxpayers and the state's medical assistance program" for providing healthcare for her two sons [24].
> Source: "Struggling Hopkins Workers Need Better Wages, Not Unusable Benefits," *The Baltimore Sun,* April 15, 2014.

Asking low-wage workers to "get an education" so they can qualify for a job that gives them respect and financial reward presupposes that the key roles workers currently play in the daily work of running our institutions is meaningless and not valuable. Wage increases don't fully address persistent structural inequality, given the low starting point and the impact of inflation. Observers noted that the 2000 Johns Hopkins employees won't exactly be "flush with cash" [25].[5] To stay afloat, many work a second job and pool their income with other family members while hoping that job loss, eviction, illness, death, or an unexpected life event doesn't occur.

Benefits place the promise of the American dream within reach of ordinary workers. They are key mechanisms to convert dead-end jobs into an entry point to a genuine career ladder. Leon Davis, 1199's founding president, conceptualized the "Funds" as organizations 100% funded by employer contributions that provide a

---

[5] Even in 1969, workers like Mrs. Mozell Smith, a 50-year-old food preparer at Hospital for Joint Diseases, recognized that winning $107 a week is "not a lot of money, but it's a lot if you're used to getting $65" [14].

range of services to union members based on terms in the negotiated contract. Funds have been replicated across many unions since. These examples are largely from 1199's contract with the League of Voluntary Hospitals and Nursing Homes based in New York City [26].[6]

- *National Benefit Fund (healthcare and pensions)* – The Fund receives employer contributions that finance the administration of services ensuring no out-of-pocket costs for medical and dental care and prescriptions. When the cost of healthcare is shifted onto employees, workers find themselves with healthcare in name only.[7] Pensions ensure that workers receive benefits in addition to their social security earnings when they retire.
- *Training and Upgrading Fund (education)* – Created in 1969 as the first of its kind in the nation, this Fund ensures access to no- or low-cost continuing education with supportive counseling, scholarships, and tuition support for high school diplomas, college degrees, certificates, and licenses. It has been replicated in union contracts in many industries across the country. Today, the Fund is training members for new positions, such as patient navigators, care coordinators, and community health workers.
- *Job Security Fund (layoffs)* – In anticipation of massive layoffs in the 1980s, 1199 created a service to give laid off workers a means to provide for their families, while they receive counseling and classes to find another job in the industry.
- *Child Care Fund* – Noticing rising child care costs, members negotiated the creation of new Fund to furnish low-cost access to summer camps, college scholarships, and youth mentoring services for their children.
- *Homeownership and Citizenship Classes* – Administered by the Training Fund, the classes coach and support people through all the stages of obtaining a mortgage and/or US citizenship.
- *Labor-Management Committees* – Workers and supervisors jointly identify projects that simplify operations and improve patient care through hundreds of successful projects that result in millions in savings. Dedicated staff train committee members in collaboration, communication, and problem-solving.

Negotiated benefits combat the structural deficits workers face. They convert jobs defined by a constant state of economic precarity into avenues for moderate stability. But most workplaces are not unionized, or workers lack the power to threaten a strike, which has been the only effective way to make gains at scale. Recognizing that all workers – not just union members – face structural challenges, most unions join coalitions to increase standards for all workers by supporting new minimum wage laws, health and safety regulations, universal pre-K, disability rights, family medical leave laws (paid and unpaid), and, of course, universal healthcare.

---

[6] To learn more, visit www.1199seiubenefits.org/.

[7] Evelyn Harris, an emergency room liaison at Niagara Falls Memorial Hospital in Buffalo, NY reported: "Fifty percent of our service and maintenance workers at Niagara Falls Memorial [Hospital] go without healthcare coverage because they can't afford it." "Profits Before Patients: Many HMOs earn billions while cutting services and increasing premiums." *1199SEIU Our Life and Times.* May 2007: 7.

Despite the pain of the historic New York City strikes, hospital leaders belatedly acknowledged that unionization reduced employee turnover, increased worker pride, and raised performance standards. They admitted: "Many...work stoppages relate to actions of unwise supervisors. All supervisors have had either to respond to training in supervisory practices or be fired" [27]. Observers noted that, "Hospitals now retain personnel experts and improve their whole approach to human relations, to the benefit of patients as well as workers" [14].

Challenge: Ignoring the Impact on Patient Care

Caring for patients is not over when your shift ends
Home Health Aide Melisa Saigo notes, "[their] life is in our hands; we can't just leave when our shift is over… but often we only get paid the flat rate even if we work longer…" [28].
    Source: Interview with Sandi Vito, April 2017.

Allied healthcare workers interact with patients at moments of deep vulnerability. Nurse aides, orderlies, and others listen to patients, console them, and respond to their needs while cleaning, bathing, feeding, and monitoring them. These workers receive a clear message that the "emotional labor of chatting, sharing stories, spending time, and being a friend" is not important. It is "not reflected in job descriptions, supported by administrators, taught in training, or rewarded in pay." Nor is it considered "billable" on official charts [29]. Nurses find difficult work conditions where they take orders from doctors and do more "'paper care than patient care'" [29].

Today workers feel coerced to give their time to preserve the dignity of patients. Unrealistic workloads mean time runs out, while workers are in the middle of bathing a client, doing laundry, or buying groceries. Workers face the moral burden of deciding whether to "'dip into the well of their own humanity to offset budget constraints and stifling rulebooks'" by staying late and arriving early to meet patient needs [29, 30].

Response: From Workers to Partners in Care

Frontline workers are best positioned to teach and foster social medicine
Lloyd Conliffe, Care Manager in Brooklyn and 1199 member, reported that the care coordination team found that, "If you don't have anywhere to sleep, you won't go to the doctor." But it took time for "doctors [and medical students] to understand the social parts of medicine" – the idea that family, social supports, and housing are important parts of health [31].
    Source: Interview with Sandi Vito, January 2017.

Inadequate staffing ratios are a long-standing problem. Undervalued work and chronic understaffing also fuels rushed, harried, neglectful, and rude care. In addition, workers easily find their ideas and insights are not welcomed or valued. One vehicle 1199 institutionalized to address this lack of voice is the Labor-Management Committee. As a result, allied health workers can be recognized as partners who address structural barriers in healthcare by using their ability to connect with patients' lives. Two examples highlight the result of promising initiatives that address structural barriers in healthcare by engaging workers' ability to connect with patients' lives.

- *Care Managers in Brooklyn, NY.* The Brooklyn Health Home project at Maimonides Medical Hospital seeks to improve health outcomes in 11 zip codes. In the newly created role of Care Manager, allied health workers function as advocates who "show people where to get assistance and how to navigate systems, as well as teaching patients to advocate for themselves" [31]. Care Managers identified housing as a healthcare issue and shared it with the care team, community networks, and testified at public hearings. Initially, doctors failed to recognize the value of health coaching, coordination of care, and connections to social services to address housing and other problems. But relationships strengthened over time, and key physicians began to educate others about the importance of housing to improving care.
- *Community Health Workers in Bronx, NY.* Bronx-Lebanon Hospital's Family Medicine Program recognizes that patients live in an interconnected web of family and neighborhood dynamics that are influenced by community organizations as well as city, state, and federal policies [32]. The project reaches patients not engaged in primary care and increases follow-up by current patients. Newly designated community health workers helped residents identify the priorities that would improve health, and then they built linkages with over 20 organizations that could address identified needs. A range of programs resulted, including youth leadership development and arts internships, exercise classes, healthy living groups, and senior citizen art groups. The Apprenticeship Program creates a meaningful entry point and career ladder and reflects a deep partnership between the union and employers [32, 33].[8]

It remains to be seen whether these pilot projects will remain small-scale experiments or function as beachheads that grow into large-scale programs that alter the mainstream experience of care.

---

[8] See Destina Garcia's story profiled by Kevin Carey in *The New York Times.* The Apprenticeship Program is a partnership between 1199SEIU Training and Employment Funds, Bronx-Lebanon Hospital Center, 1199SEIU United Healthcare Workers East, LaGuardia Community College, and the New York Alliance for Careers in Healthcare. "Trump's Apprentice Plan Seems to Need a Mentor," Kevin Carey September 28, 2017. https://nyti.ms/2yuszuY.

Key Learnings: Agents, Allies, and Mavericks Seeking Structural Change

Charity has its limits

The Baltimore Sun observed, "Johns Hopkins University has been at the vanguard of efforts to improve East Baltimore through charitable work, so why not start with health care workers?" [23].

Source: "A Win-Win for Hopkins," Editorial, *The Baltimore Sun*, July 8, 2014.

For social, cultural, economic, and historic reasons, the healthcare industry – like many other employers – takes the low road with their employees, maximizing income at the expense of individual and societal health. Unionization is the exception. More often charity, benevolence and philanthropy reign. But those approaches have not reduced structural inequalities for healthcare workers at scale. Nor has heartfelt appeals to justice, fairness, and rights. Rising through the ranks by acquiring more degrees and certificates has not been an effective strategy for many workers. The rungs in the ladder of educational opportunity are broken, leaving many debt-ridden and underemployed. Overall, offering individual rewards to "good" and "deserving" workers does not address structural inequality.

Workers acting as "agents of change" through unions and broad based social movements have been the most effective driver of large-scale change that reduces structural inequality. In 2018, nurses at Johns Hopkins Medicine and graduate students at Johns Hopkins University pursued unionization [34, 35]. Collective actions – such as marches, rallies, lawsuits, social media campaigns, and, as a last resort, work stoppages – have been necessary but not sufficient.

Allies are critical. In the 1950s and 1960s, donations from other unions, neighbors, churches, and supportive organizations allowed workers to avoid starvation and homelessness during strikes. Allies – especially governors and other elected officials – also exerted pressure on employers to urge them to settle [10, 13]. For example, Martin Luther King, Jr. called New York's Governor Nelson Rockefeller to urge him to keep his promise to repeal the law that made hospital worker strikes illegal [13]. Smaller actions count, such as the letter of support for striking workers signed by Johns Hopkins physicians and published in *The Baltimore Sun* [36].

Mavericks also help. Typically, trustees resist changing their employment practices and prefer to rationalize the ongoing poverty of allied healthcare workers [37]. Sometimes, maverick board members disagreed with their peers and took public stances. For example, Dr. Martin Cherkasky, CEO of Montefiore Hospital in the Bronx (New York), was shunned by colleagues after persuading the board to permit hospital unionization in 1958 [38]. Influential Congressman Emanuel Celler resigned from a hospital board because they authorized arrests of striking workers [10]. Perhaps a new generation of clinicians and healthcare leaders will spearhead an approach where the industry no longer generates the very inequalities it subsequently "treats."

Application: Building Alliances with Healthcare Workers for Structural Change

The healthcare industry is not unique in its reliance on society's low-wage structures as central to its financial and care delivery models. Industry leaders can learn to see and transform the inherited hierarchies of class, race, gender, and status *within* medical settings. Collaborations with allied healthcare workers will be essential to achieve fairness and health at scale.

1. *See workers holistically and cultivate genuine partnerships.* Forging effective partnerships with healthcare workers can be a key component of achieving structural competence and system transformation. Workers are also patients, family members, community leaders, advocates, taxpayers, neighbors, and voters. Healthcare workers are deeply invested in ending the perversities that plague our healthcare system and our society. Creating meaningful patient, worker, and community collaborations at scale is new to the industry. To avoid superficial engagement, healthcare organizations must partner with experienced entities like labor unions and grassroots groups with a track record of building community-based partnerships with healthcare entities (see, examples at www.community-catalyst.org or www.interactioninstitute.org). The presumption that those with the most resources have the best or most appropriate answers must be set aside for real engagement with those who work on the front lines.

2. *Reinvest savings to cultivate community and population health.* As the country with the most expensive healthcare system and the worst health outcomes, savings are both possible and necessary. The ideas of patients, workers, and communities can lead to significant savings and improvements. When workers' ideas make a difference, institutions should share the rewards, not just the burdens of problem-solving. Savings should be reinvested to support and cultivate healthy patients, workers, and communities. Furthermore, better patient care at lower cost should not occur at the expense of workers who have benefited least from the industry's wealth. Too often the search for savings perpetuates historic inequities as financial pressures lead institutions to squeeze workers at the bottom of the hierarchy to compensate for inefficiencies generated by the fragmented fee-for-service system [39, 40].

3. *Guarantee free healthcare for all healthcare workers.* Eliminate high co-pays and deductibles for employees in the healthcare sector. With over 200,000 members in New York City, our data shows they also suffer from chronic healthcare problems (heart disease, diabetes, high blood pressure). Allied health workers often work at the expense of their own health. In addition, other possible interventions by employers include substantive health and wellness of their employees. In addition, they can forgive the medical debt of their low-wage employees. Employers can also voluntarily divulge the number of employees receiving public health insurance and social assistance.[9]

---

[9] See Walker, Andrea K. 2014. "Union wants hospitals to disclose employees on public assistance." *The Baltimore Sun.* May 21. www.baltimoresun.com/health/blog/bs-hs-union-hscrc-20140521-story.html.

4. *Support organizations and policies that improve the lives of all workers.* Speak out in big and small ways on the connection between a good job and good health. Support structural interventions such as affordable housing, paid sick days and family leave for all, universal pre-K and child care, a $15 minimum wage and pay equity, climate justice and disability rights, anti-violence and anti-police brutality initiatives, and universal education and healthcare. Fair access to the structure of opportunity is essential. Through unions and alliances with other social movements, healthcare workers forced systemic changes that gave working families a chance at the American dream.

Acknowledgments   Heartfelt thanks to Sandi Vito (Executive Director, 1199SEIU Training and Employment Funds) who conducted interviews with 1199SEIU members, Lloyd Conliffe and Melisa Saigo. Sandi, along with Yvonne Armstrong (1199SEIU Senior Executive Vice President for Long Term Care), provided critical early support and feedback. Barbara Caress's erudition on health policy and 1199 history is unsurpassed, and she guided me to the Health Policy Advisory Center archives. Virginia Eubanks, Heidi Hamilton, and Catherine McLaren also provided close readings and insights.

Appendix

In the Classroom

We need healthcare practitioners with the skill to build a robust and just health system. Classroom activities can include:

- *Guest speakers*: To build awareness of workforce relations and the social dimensions of medical care. Seek multiple perspectives on the same issue.
  - *Unions and worker organizations*: Their elected officers, activist workers, and their policy, research, communications, and organizing staffs can offer valuable perspectives. For worker experiences, arrange for guest speakers (workers need an honorarium for these visits) or create "a day in their shoes" experiences shadowing community health workers, home care workers, and other key allied health workers. Use documentaries and videos to bring worker experiences into the classroom.
  - *Worker organizations*: Home care worker growth outpaces all other categories in the next decade. The national campaign, Caring Across Generations, seeks to build a true system of affordable long-term care and build a culture of care.
  - *Training funds*: They critically analyze industry trends and work with both management and labor to offer relevant interventions. See, for example, www.1199seiubenefits.org.
  - *Employer and industry organizations*: They negotiate with unions and represent multiple employers. In New York City, it is the League of Voluntary Hospitals and Homes (www.lvhh.com) and the Greater New York Hospital Association (www.gnyha.org/).

- *Administrators*: Their mindsets and decisions affect thousands of workers and patients. Include "middle managers" responsible for implementation on the ground.
- *Trailblazers*: Institutions that have implemented innovative workforce or care delivery changes at scale, like Kaiser Permanente.
- *Network and capacity builders*: Building a better future for healthcare with community partners takes deep skill to avoid typical pitfalls and to identify grounded and sustainable innovations. Ideas, resources, and tools are available from www.communitycatalyst.org/ and www.interactioninstitute.org/.
- *Academics*: To build a conceptual vocabulary and critical analysis that integrates historical, economic, and sociological dynamics with healthcare delivery. See the citations in the "Agents of Change" chapter.
- *Patients*: To excavate the range of interactions they have beyond the clinical encounter. In addition, seek nursing home and home care patients as well to engage questions of continuity of care and of the social factors that influence the receipt of care and adherence to treatment plans.

• *Historical cases*:
  - *Johns Hopkins Medical Center Strike 1969 and 2014*
    Video of Annie Henry talking about Coretta Scott King at Johns Hopkins strike in 1969. http://hardshipathopkins.org/coretta-scott-king-at-hopkins/ 2014 accounts of the Johns Hopkins strike. Available at www.hardshipathopkins.org
  - *1969 Hospital Strike in Charleston, SC*
    Documentary: *I Am Somebody* (30 min), directed by Madeline Anderson, a trailblazing African American female director. http://icarusfilms.com/if-iams Primary sources including audio clips of interviews – http://ldhi.library.cofc. edu/exhibits/show/charleston_hospital_workers_mo/sources_3
  - *Health Policy Advisory Center*
    From 1968 to 1994, the Health Policy Advisory Center provided critical analysis of the medical industrial complex, a term they coined. Their articles and books investigate the industry's structure as well as grassroots community-based efforts to combat inequality. There archives are accessible and searchable online at www.healthpacbulletin.org.
    Cartoons on the healthcare industry by award-winning illustrator Bill Plympton www.healthpacbulletin.org/wp-content/uploads/2013/02/H-PAC-Bill-Plympton-Drawings-Scanned_007.png
  - *Podcast on history of Bellevue Hospital as almshouse hospital* – http://boweryboys.libsyn.com/-152-bellevue-hospital
• *Read healthcare worker contracts*: Learn the concerns of workers and the benefits and protections negotiated. For example, see 1199SEIU's master contract with the League of Voluntary Hospitals and Homes of New York at lvhh.com/current-agreements/.
• *Write accessible pieces like letters to the editor and op-eds*: Choose an issue and write it. Sending is optional but practicing helps. Given today's technology, op-docs, blogs, and other vehicles for sharing perspectives also matter. See, for example, "Invisible Colleagues" by Benjamin Oldfield, MD in *The New England*

Journal of Medicine August 27, 2015. www.nejm.org/doi/full/10.1056/
NEJMp1506873.

- *Awareness and reflection*: It's disturbing and disruptive to learn we have blinders. Build awareness and the capacity to hold uncomfortable truths and contradictions via workshops and exercises with partner organizations dedicated to such learning. Class action's workshops and resources on class (classism.org) and racial justice trainings (this is not diversity training) (https://www.raceforward.org/trainings; http://interactioninstitute.org/trainings/).

References

1. Vail B. Striking workers shame prestigious Johns Hopkins hospital over low pay [Internet]. In: In These Times. 2014 April 10 [cited 2017 Dec 3]. Available from: http://inthese-times.com/working/entry/16541/striking_workers_shame_prestigious_johns_hopkins_hospital_over_low_pay
2. Centers for Medicare and Medicaid Services (US). Historical national health expenditure data [Internet]. Washington, DC. 2018 Jan. Available at https://www.cms.gov/research-statistics-data-and-systems/statistics-trends-and-reports/nationalhealthexpenddata/national-healthaccountshistorical.html
3. Glenn EN. Forced to care: coercion and caregiving in America. Cambridge: Harvard University Press; 2012. p. 272.
4. Gascon C. US healthcare and future job growth [Internet]. St. Louis: Federal Reserve Bank of St. Louis. 2018 May 21 [cited 2018 Sep 15]. Available from: https://www.stlouisfed.org/on-the-economy/2018/may/health-care-future-job-growth
5. Hartocollis A. Bellevue Marks 275 years of taking care. The New York Times. 2011. Dec 15.
6. Wall BM. History of hospitals [Internet]. Philadelphia: University of Pennsylvania School of Nursing. Nd [cited 2017 June 25]. Available from: www.nursing.upenn.edu/nhhc/nurses-institutions-caring/history-of-hospitals/index.php
7. Foundation Aiding the Elderly. The history of nursing homes [Internet]. Nd [cited 2017 June 25]. Available from: http://www.4fate.org/history.pdf
8. Eubanks V. Automating inequality: how high-tech tools profile, police, and punish the poor. New York: St. Martin's Press; 2018. 265p.
9. Knights Jr. M.D., EM. Bellevue hospital. History magazine [Internet]. Issue 2. Nd [cited 2017 Dec 3]. Available from: www.history-magazine.com/bellevue.html
10. Pritchett WE. A northern civil rights movement: community race relations in Brooklyn and the beth-el hospital strike of 1962. Labor's Heritage. 2000;10(Fall/Winter):4.
11. Hirsh J, Beka D. The first hundred years of the mount sinai hospital of New York, 1852–1952 [Internet]. New York: Random House. 1952 [cited 2017 June 25]. Available from: https://archive.org/stream/firsthundredyear1952jose/firsthundredyear1952jose_djvu.txt
12. Weissman E. Non-profit hospitals and labor unions. 8 Cleveland-Marshall Law Review 482. 1959 [cited 2017 June 5]. Available from: www.engagedscholarship.csuohio.edu/clevstlrev
13. Fink L, Greenberg B. Upheaval in the quiet zone: 1199SEIU and the politics of healthcare unionism. Urbana: University of Illinois Press; 2009. second edition [1989]. 392p.
14. Raskin AH. A union with a 'soul'. The New York Times. 1970 Mar 22 [cited 2017 June 1]. Available from: https://nyti.ms/1H0fqYm.
15. Health Policy Advisory Center. Hospital unions: a long time coming. In: Health/PAC Bulletin. 1970 July–August. New York: Health Policy Advisory Center. Available from: www.health-pacbulletin.org.
16. Boris E, Klein J. Labor on the home front: unionizing home-based care workers. New Labor Forum 2008 Summer. 17(2): 32–41.

17. Caress B. Home is where the patients are: New York home care workers' contract victory. Health/PAC Bulletin 1988 Fall 18(3). 4–14. Health Policy Advisory Center.
18. Flack A. 50 who carried the 1199 torch: profiles of our pioneers. In: Our life and times: a journal of 1199SEIU. New York: 1199SEIU; 2009.
19. Mount Sinai 150th Anniversary Committee. 1852–2002: the sesquicentennial [Internet]. New York: Mount Sinai Hospital: New York. 2002 [cited 2017 May 31]. Available from: https://icahn.mssm.edu/files/ISMMS/Assets/About%20the%20School/Academic%20IT%20 (AIT)/Levy%20Library/Sesquicentennial.pdf
20. Peterson RR. Balancing priorities and resources at Johns Hopkins [Internet]. Commentary/ Op-ed. Baltimore Sun. 2014 Apr 11 [cited 2017 Dec 3]. Available from: http://www.baltimoresun.com/news/opinion/oped/bs-ed-jh-labor-dispute-20140410-story.html
21. Williams IV JJ. Thousands gather to protest pay at Hopkins hospital [Internet]. Baltimore Sun. 2014 May 10 [cited 2017 Dec 3]. Available from: http://www.baltimoresun.com/health/bs-md-hopkins-protest-20140510-story.html
22. McFadden RD. Leon Davis, 85, Head of Health-Care Union, Dies [Internet]. New York Times. 1992 Sep15 [cited 2017 June 22].
23. Baltimore Sun. A win-win for Hopkins [Internet]. Editorial. 2014 July 8 [cited 2017 June 4]. Available from: http://www.baltimoresun.com/news/opinion/editorial/bs-ed-hopkins-20140708-story.html
24. Robbins K. Struggling Hopkins workers need better wages, not unusable benefits [Internet]. Letter to the Editor. Baltimore Sun. 2014 April 15 [cited 2017 June 13]. Available from: http://www.baltimoresun.com/news/opinion/readersrespond/bs-ed-hopkins-worker-letter-20140415-story.html
25. Reutter M. Victor in Hopkins labor dispute is not your granddaddy's union [Internet]. Baltimore Brew. 2014 July 8 [cited 2017 June 3]. Available from: https://www.baltimorebrew.com/2014/07/08/victor-in-hopkins-labor-dispute-is-not-your-grandaddys-union/
26. Hudson G, Caress B. New York's 1199 in 1989: rebuilding a troubled union. Labor Research Review. 1991;1(17):6.
27. North D, Foner M. Celebrating the life of Leon Davis. New York: 1199 New York's Health and Hospitals Union. (Publication for Davis' memorial tribute at Lincoln Center's Avery Fischer Hall.) 1992 Oct 5. P. 19 On file with author.
28. Saigo, M. Interview. Home Health Aide and 1199 member. 2017 April. (Interviewed by Sandi Vito).
29. Ducey A. Never good enough: health care workers and the false promise of job training. New York: Cornell ILR Press; 2008.
30. Boris E, Klein J. Frontline caregivers: still struggling. Dissent Magazine. 2017 Spring.
31. Conliffe, L. Interview. Care Manager and 1199 member. 2017 January. (Interviewed by Sandi Vito).
32. Findley S, Sergio M, Hicks A. et al. community health worker integration into the health team accomplishes the triple aim in a patient-centered medical home: a Bronx tale. Jnl Amb Care Mgmt 2014 (37):82–91. Available from: http://www.blhfamilymed.com/Scholarly-Activity/presentations-posters-and-conventions
33. Carey K. Trump's apprentice plan seems to need a mentor. New York Times. 2017 Sep 28 [cited 2017 Dec 3]. Available from: https://nyti.ms/2yuszuY
34. McDaniels AK. Some Johns Hopkins nurses trying to unionize. Baltimore Sun. 2018 Mar 19.
35. Richman T. Johns Hopkins graduate students announce unionization plans [Internet]. Baltimore Sun. 2018 Sep 26 [cited 2018 Oct 2]. Available from: http://www.baltimoresun.com/news/maryland/education/higher-ed/bs-md-ci-hopkins-union-20180926-story.html
36. Nayak Z, et al. Hopkins should support its employees [Internet]. Letter to the Editor. Baltimore Sun. 2014 April 7 [cited 2018 Oct 2]. Available from: http://www.baltimoresun.com/news/opinion/bs-ed-hopkins-letter-20140407-story.html

37. Frank T. Straight into the fox news buzzsaw: why elite, billionaire liberalism always backfires [Internet]. Salon. 2014 April 20 [cited 2017 Aug 2]. Available from: www.salon.com
38. Halbfinger DM. Dr. Martin Cherkasky, 85; led expansion of Montefiore. New York Times. 1997 September 8.
39. Clark C. Berwick Names 11 Monsters Facing Hospital Industry [Internet]. Health Leaders Media. 2013 July 29.
40. Gawande A. Big Med. New Yorker. 2012 August 13.

Physicians as Policy Advocates: From the Clinic to the State House

Julie Netherland

The Challenge

Though few clinicians are trained on how to influence policy, the policy environment has an enormous impact on patient health. Government policies – whether federal, state, or municipal – shape everything from the delivery of healthcare to the patient's physical and social environment. From insurance reimbursement to food quality and access to clean air and water, health is affected daily by the decisions of policymakers. Another policy arena that profoundly impacts health – one that should be of great concern to medical providers – is drug policy. Historically, battles over drug policy have been framed by two, often competing, ideologies: one which sees drug use a moral failing and a crime that should be punished and another which sees it as an illness or disease requiring compassion and treatment. The question of who "owns" the problem of drug use – law enforcement or medicine – has been debated for decades. More recently, harm reduction – an approach that seeks to minimize the harms associated with drug use and our drug policies – has gained some traction. Because they are well respected, knowledgeable, highly credentialed, and can speak directly to the impact of policies on their patients, the voices of physicians as drug policy advocates are both powerful and desperately needed. Unfortunately, few physicians are equipped or have the time to engage in policy advocacy. Can physicians become effective policy advocates? And if so, how?

This chapter describes how one advocacy organization, the Drug Policy Alliance (DPA), works with physicians and researchers to reform drug policies. By describing the involvement of physicians in three different drug policy reform campaigns,

J. Netherland (✉)
Drug Policy Alliance, New York City, NY, USA
e-mail: jnetherland@drugpolicy.org

© Springer Nature Switzerland AG 2019
H. Hansen, J. M. Metzl (eds.), *Structural Competency in Mental Health and Medicine*,
https://doi.org/10.1007/978-3-030-10525-9_17

this chapter illustrates how physicians can improve the health of their patients and thousands of others by changing the policy landscape. It also discusses the challenges that physicians may face in becoming advocates and offers suggestions for overcoming those challenges.

Framework

Traditionally, clinicians have been trained to deal with addiction at the level of the individual, offering medication-assisted treatments, counseling, and/or referrals to treatment. Often understood as chronic relapsing brain disease, clinicians and policymakers alike seldom consider how structural determinants affect decisions to use substances, severity of use, access to treatment and resources to deal with addiction, and the systems that intervene when someone choses to buy, use or sell drugs. In a country like the USA, where drug policy is largely driven by ideology, one's social location deeply affects one's experiences of drugs and of the criminal justice apparatus that has been built to deal with "drug problems." For example, one's race and neighborhood can profoundly affect whether drug use is treated as an illness or as a crime. A structural competency approach to drug policy allows clinicians to look through the lens of social and political context to better understand all the forces that impact their patients, including how the war on drugs and the stigmatization and criminalization of people who use drugs impacts health and wellness. Moreover, clinicians are well positioned to influence drug policy in ways that can increase their reach beyond individual patients.

Since Nixon declared the War on Drugs in 1973, most of US drug policy has been largely driven by a "law and order" strategy that has resulted in the mass incarceration of millions of people, primarily Black and Brown men. These policies disproportionately affect low income and communities of color through racially biased policing, spatially concentrated incarceration, and the host of collateral consequences associated with a drug arrest, all of which can cause significant disruptions in the health of families, communities, and individuals. Other drug policies – such as the provision of buprenorphine, access to medical marijuana, and availability of harm reduction services for people who use drugs – can improve patient health.

The Drug Policy Alliance is a national, nonprofit advocacy organization working to end the war on drugs and move the nation's drug policies away from an approach grounded in criminal toward one rooted in public health approach. Committed to evidence-based policy, DPA works closely with researchers, clinicians, and other experts to try and bridge the divide between research and policy. While we understand that policy is driven by many factors other than research, we remain committed to basing our policy campaigns on the best possible evidence about what works. Our philosophy is that the most effective policies are those born from a coalition between those directly impacted by the policies, advocacy, and service organizations working on the issue and experts in the field, such as researchers and clinicians.

The Path

Medical providers, whether in engage in research or patient care, have an important role to play in many of the issues on which we work. Moreover, given the growing understanding of addiction as a medical issue and the failure of punitive approaches, policymakers are more ready than ever to listen to medical providers on the issue of drug policy. Many lawmakers understand the impact of drug policy on health, and because of their training and credentials, physicians often have credibility with policymakers.

While most physicians have received little if any training on how to do policy advocacy, DPA is able to quickly provide the skills needed, demystify the political process, offer a grounding in the particular political jurisdiction and its dynamics, and create avenues for physicians to engage effectively given the limitations on their time and capacity. Physicians can play a number of roles, but among the valuable assets they bring to advocacy work are their "real-world" experience and stories about how policies affect patient health (i.e., humanizing the issue), credentials and training, and expertise and their ability to translate research into lay language accessible to policymakers and the public.

One example of how physicians can humanize an issue is the role they played during a campaign to legalize medical marijuana in New York in 2014. Six hundred and fifty New York physicians signed up to be part of New York Physicians for Compassionate Care (NYPCC), a group dedicated to insuring that medical marijuana would be available as one tool to better treat their patients. Working with DPA, physicians from NYPCC, helped bring the issue to life by sharing patient stories at press conferences, during meetings with legislators, and through "doctor profiles," short vignettes explaining a doctor's interest in medical marijuana and how to it could benefit his/her patients. Physicians also played a crucial role in presenting research about medical marijuana's efficacy to lawmakers and answering their questions about the medical use of cannabis and its potential risks.

When the law passed in 2014, the program was small, narrow, cost-prohibitive, and bureaucratically cumbersome as a result of political compromises. Physicians continued to work closely with DPA advocating for improvements and expansions to the program. However, the New York legislature had moved on and was less interested in improving access to medical marijuana than they were in addressing the opioid overdose crisis. Fortunately, one physician-researcher with whom we worked had published an important study showing that states with medical marijuana programs had significantly lower rates of opioid overdose deaths. We worked with the researcher to publish an op-ed, submit testimony, and call key legislators with the goal of adding severe, chronic pain as a condition that would qualify one to participate in the medical marijuana program. A few months after these efforts, New York did add chronic pain to the program, potentially helping thousands of suffering patients. The key to this success was using a pivotal piece of research strategically to take advantage of the political concern of the day – providing an alternative to opioid analgesics. In intervening at the policy level, this physician-researcher helped expand the medical marijuana program to patients in need and potentially reduce the use of and overdose from unnecessary opioids.

Using a structural competency framework, physicians can not only help respond to a political moment but also identify and initiate policy improvements of their own. In meetings with physicians working with people who use drugs, we discovered that one barrier to treatment was the practice of insurance companies requiring prior authorization before allowing the prescription of buprenorphine, a medication to treat opioid addiction. According to the physicians with whom we worked, prior authorization was both causing patients to needlessly relapse while waiting for the approval to go through and discouraging physicians from prescribing buprenorphine because they did not have the time or inclination to hassle with the insurance companies. Even those willing to do so were reporting that significant amounts of their time were devoted to prior authorization paperwork rather than patient care. Acting on this information, we worked with the physician who first identified the issue and legislators in Albany to draft a bill that would eliminate the requirement for prior authorization. In an unusual move for drug policy reform legislation, which is generally carried by progressive lawmakers, we approached a senate Republican about sponsoring the bill. After explaining how access to buprenorphine could help address the opioid problem in his community – an issue of grave concern to his constituents – he agreed to champion the bill, making it easier for us to garner other Republican support. We then worked with the physician to publish an op-ed explaining the problem in lay terms, which we distributed to every member of the legislature. Following a series of meetings with key influencers in Albany, the bill was passed and signed into law. The key to the success of this effort was timing and securing bipartisan support; we presented the issue at a time with policymakers from both parties who were struggling to address the opioid overdose crisis and needed a political win. Instead of continuing to intervene with each individual who needed prior authorization, by focusing on the policy barrier, we were able to enact structural change with the promise of improving access for all buprenorphine patients.

Sometimes, as in the two examples above, going directly to the legislature makes sense. Other times an issue is so new or controversial that the strategic move is to generate a public discussion and support before legislation is filed. This was our approach in advancing safer consumption spaces. A safer consumption space (sometimes known as a safe injection facility) provides safe, clean place for people to use drugs, usually under medical supervision. In operation for decades in Europe and Canada, a large body of research has shown the efficacy of drug consumption rooms in reducing overdose deaths and the transmission of blood-borne diseases while linking a hard-to-reach population to needed services and treatment. Despite the evidence of their success, they have never been implemented in the USA and, until recently, were considered too controversial to even discuss as a viable strategy. However, as the opioid crisis worsened and spread to white, suburban communities, more harm reduction strategies, like safe consumption spaces, started to be considered. In New York, when the idea was first introduced, it had surprising amount of support among the public and the media. However, one conservative lawmaker, who opposed them, told a news outlet that no clinician would ever support such an approach. Within days, a physician had drafted a sign-on letter and obtained the signatures of almost 100 physicians in New York declaring their support for safe consumption spaces. Physicians have also joined a coalition of advocacy groups and people who currently or formerly used drugs to push for a drug consumption room in New York and have published op-eds explaining how drug consumption rooms would help their patients. These physicians understood that the public consumption of drugs has to do with structural issues, such as homelessness, and was putting their patients at risk for law enforcement involvement, overdose, and other sequelae of rushed and dirty injections such as abscesses and blood-borne illnesses. In this case, physicians played an essential role in countering the opposition and helping to frame and own the narrative about the issue. Rather than letting policymakers or the press speak on their behalf, they proactively organized themselves to promote a different message about what was best for their patients.

Key Learnings

These three examples illustrate just some of the ways physicians can influence policy – from low-threshold activities, such as signing onto a petition or letter, to more involved engagement, such as conceptualizing and lobbying for the passage of new legislation. Generally speaking, policy change can be glacially slow; it can take years to pass even incremental reform. While the chief indicator of success is the passage of a bill or change in policy, a policy campaign often has important effects that are difficult to measure, such as reframing an issue, changing the terms of the debate, or engaging a group of people in political action who have not previously been engaged. Therefore, in addition to looking at bills passed and signed into law as an indicator of change, we also look at transformational metrics, such as how the media is reporting on our issues; how legislators speak about "controversial" issues, such as safe consumption spaces; or how many new people met with their legislators about drug policy. Shaping the narrative, educating the public and lawmakers, and owning the issue are critical precursors to policy change. Physicians have important roles to play in the lives of their individual patients, but as these examples illustrate, they can also influence structural and policy-level changes.

While our work engaging physicians in policy reform efforts has been successful, it comes with some challenges. Both physicians and researchers face a number of barriers in doing advocacy. The biggest issues are time and competing priorities. Very few physicians have institutional incentives for being more politically engaged and are usually doing this work on top of all their other responsibilities. Some physician-researchers are concerned that their political advocacy gives them the appearance of bias, though many understand the critical importance of political engagement. Another difficulty is the timeframe for action. While it can take forever to change policy, when policy proposals do start to move, they move quickly. This can mean that the need for information or for a physician to weigh-in can be immediate or within a few hours. For busy physicians, meeting the narrow window of opportunity can prove challenging. In addition, there is often a mismatch in language. Many physicians, especially those who are also researchers, understandably want to express information carefully with precision and nuance. Unfortunately, most policymakers, like the media, are dealing with thousands of different issues and priorities and want the sound-bite version of the idea expressed. Bridging this gap can be difficult. Fortunately, the problem of language and making information accessible can be taught, and many physicians have a natural inclination for it since they often communicate complex information to patients and families.

Perhaps one of the biggest barriers for anyone hoping to influence policy is mystification of political process. Most legislatures have arcane procedures and rituals, and a great deal of policy work relies on personal relationships and understanding the power dynamics at play at any given time on a particular issue. The easiest way for physicians to engage in policy change efficiently and effectively is to partner with a policy organization that understands the political dynamics, personalities, and issues confronting a given jurisdiction. This requires doing a little research to find out what advocacy organizations are working on the issues of concern and what their track record of success is.

The Office of Academic Engagement (OAE) at the Drug Policy Alliance was founded, in large part, to provide clinicians and researchers with the tools they need to engage in effective policy advocacy. OAE works one-on-one with and offers trainings for clinicians and researchers on how policy really gets made, their role in shaping policy, how to engage in the political process, and how to make their work accessible to the media and to policymakers. In addition, OAE offers a series of webinars to support this work on topics ranging from how to write an op-ed and knowledge translation to how to use social media to shape public discourse.

Other Situations

Physicians should not be expected to be experts on the policymaking process, but, nonetheless, they have a critical role to play. There is no doubt that policy affects the health of individuals, families, and communities and that intervening at the policy level has the potential to improve (or harm) the health of thousands. The skills and actions described above have applicability beyond drug policy and could be applied to other reform efforts. Physicians are well poised to identify the structural factors that impact their patients' health. Addressing many of these will require intervening at the policy level. While engaging in the political process can seem daunting, with some modest effort, physicians can become powerful advocates for structural change.

Given the assault on our healthcare and social services system at the federal level, combined with a return to "law and order" approaches to drug policy, physician voices are especially needed now in drug policy reform efforts. Physicians are uniquely situated to help us move our nation's drug policies from an approach rooted in punishment and racism to one grounded in science, compassion, and health. In doing so, they will be improving the well-being of their patients and the rest of us.

Part V

Bibliography

Clinical Applications of Structural Competency: A Select Bibliography

Laura G. Duncan

This bibliography is a compilation of writings relevant to structural competency. Healthcare workers, researchers, and activists have long been working to identify, intervene in, and disrupt systemic oppressions related to health. While there is a wide range of scholarship on health inequalities, this bibliography focuses on articulations and applications of the principles of structural competency. Not every piece in this bibliography explicitly uses the term structural competency; in fact, many predate the use of the term. Instead, this list represents a sample of the intellectual and political inspiration for the structural competency framework and the ways that healthcare can address upstream determinants of health.

The first section of this bibliography, "Structural Competency," includes pieces that explicitly utilize the term structural competency. Many of these articles focus on medical education, which reflects that structural competency first emerged in response to "cultural competency" in the training of health professionals. These pieces describe how structural competency can offer a corrective lens for an overly narrow educational focus on individual behavior and pharmaco-technical interventions. These authors describe upstream interventions designed to produce engaged clinicians and resistance to the institutional discrimination that makes people sick.

The next section of this bibliography "From Cultural Competency to Cultural Humility," explores critiques that cultural competency, in its focus on the beliefs and behaviors of patients, may not lead to an assessment of power and inequality. This section also includes pieces that represent the emergence of the term "cultural humility," a concept that questions the idea of competency itself. Instead, cultural

L. G. Duncan (✉)
Medical Scientist Training Program, Department of Anthropology, History and Social Medicine, University of California, San Francisco, San Francisco, CA, USA
e-mail: laura.duncan@ucsf.edu

© Springer Nature Switzerland AG 2019
H. Hansen, J. M. Metzl (eds.), *Structural Competency in Mental Health and Medicine*,
https://doi.org/10.1007/978-3-030-10525-9_18

humility offers a framework that eschews the goal of expertise in regard to culture and instead centers self-reflection, collaborative learning with patients and the communities from which they come, and an acknowledgment of unequal power relations within and outside of clinical spaces.

References in the third section "Structural Determinants and Interventions: Public Health Looks Upstream" sketch how the discipline of public health has intervened on social determinants of health. This focus has also expanded, as represented by the increasing use of the phrase "the structural determinants of health," to include even more upstream, large economic, political, and institutional structures. This section also includes writing on social medicine, a movement that has long called for healthcare to engage with systemic forces with an especially rich history and contemporary practice in Latin America. There is also a subsection of articles dedicated to medical-legal partnerships. The literature on this topic explores how cross-disciplinary collaboration can provide creative solutions to upstream problems. These writings show how a structural analysis can influence the design and outcomes of public health interventions.

The final section "Advocacy and Activism: Structural Organizing in Action" highlights structural analysis and political projects. It sketches the history of advocacy and activism around structural health inequalities, from clinics run by the Black Panther Party to medical students advocating for increased abortion access. Many of these movements were student or community-led, grassroots and designed by and for those most affected. Structural competency is inspired by such movements that recognize the goal of healthcare not solely as symptom reduction, but also as promoting political representation, human rights, and freedom from violence.

Further Reading

Structural Competency

1. Bromage B, Encandela JA, Cranford M, Diaz E, Williamson B, Spell VT, et al. Understanding health disparities through the eyes of community members: a structural competency education intervention. Acad Psychiatry. 2018:1–4.
2. Conley D, Malaspina D. Socio-genomics and structural competency. J Bioeth Inq. 2016;13(2):193–202.
3. Donald CA, DasGupta S, Metzl JM, Eckstrand KL. Queer frontiers in medicine: a structural competency approach. Acad Med. 2017;92(3):345–50.
4. Downey MM, Gómez AM. Structural competency and reproductive health. AMA J Ethics. 2018;20(3):211–23.
5. Drevdahl DJ. Culture shifts: from cultural to structural theorizing in nursing. Nurs Res. 2018;67(2):146–60.
6. Hansen H, Metzl JM. Structural competency in the U.S. healthcare crisis: putting social and policy interventions into clinical practice. J Bioeth Inq. 2016;13(2):179–83.
7. Hansen H, Braslow J, Rohrbaugh RM. From cultural to structural competency—training psychiatry residents to act on social determinants of health and institutional racism. JAMA Psychiat. 2018;75(2):117–8.

8. Hansen H, Metzl JM. New medicine for the U.S. health care system: training physicians for structural interventions. Acad Med. 2017;92(3):279–81.

9. Holmes S. Fresh fruit, broken bodies: migrant farmworkers in the United States. Berkeley: University of California Press; 2013.

10. Kirmayer LJ, Kronick R, Rousseau C. Advocacy as key to structural competency in psychiatry. JAMA Psychiat. 2018;75(2):119–20.

11. Merritt R, Rougas S. Multidisciplinary approach to structural competency teaching. Med Educ. 2018;52(11):1191–2.

12. Metzl JM. The protest psychosis: how schizophrenia became a black disease. Boston: Beacon Press; 2011.

13. Metzl JM, Hansen H. Structural competency: theorizing a new medical engagement with stigma and inequality. Soc Sci Med. 2014;103:126–33.

14. Metzl JM, Hansen H. Structural competency and psychiatry. JAMA Psychiat. 2018;75(2):115–6.

15. Metzl JM, Petty J, Olowojoba OV. Using a structural competency framework to teach structural racism in pre-health education. Soc Sci Med. 2018;199:189–201.

16. Metzl JM, Petty J. Integrating and assessing structural competency in an innovative prehealth curriculum at Vanderbilt University. Acad Med. 2017;92(3):354–9.

17. Metzl JM, Roberts DE. Structural competency meets structural racism: race, politics, and the structure of medical knowledge. Virtual Mentor. 2014;16(9):674–90.

18. Neff J, Knight KR, Satterwhite S, Nelson N, Matthews J, Holmes SM. Teaching structure: a qualitative evaluation of a structural competency training for resident physicians. J Gen Intern Med. 2017;32(4):430–3.

19. Paul EG, Curran M, Tobin Tyler E. The medical-legal partnership approach to teaching social determinants of health and structural competency in residency programs. Acad Med. 2017;92(3):292–8.

20. Petty J, Metzl JM, Keys MR. Developing and evaluating an innovative structural competency curriculum for pre-health students. J Med Humanit. 2017;38(4):459–71.

21. Tsevat RK, Sinha AA, Gutierrez KJ, DasGupta S. Bringing home the health humanities: narrative humility, structural competency, and engaged pedagogy. Acad Med. 2015;90(11):1462–5.

22. Wren Serbin J, Donnelly E. The impact of racism and Midwifery's lack of racial diversity: a literature review. J Midwifery Womens Health. 2016;61(6):694–706.

From Cultural Competency to Cultural Humility

1. Angoff NR, Duncan L, Roxas N, Hansen H. Power day: addressing the use and abuse of power in medical training. J Bioeth Inq. 2016;13(2):203–13.

2. Bourgois P, Holmes SM, Sue K, Quesada J. Structural vulnerability: operationalizing the concept to address health disparities in clinical care. Acad Med. 2017;92(3):299–307.

3. Chang E -shie, Simon M, Dong X. Integrating cultural humility into health care professional education and training. Adv Health Sci Educ Theory Pract. 2012;17(2):269–78.

4. Dao DK, Goss AL, Hoekzema AS, Kelly LA, Logan AA, Mehta SD, et al. Integrating theory, content, and method to foster critical consciousness in medical students: a comprehensive model for cultural competence training. Acad Med. 2017;92(3):335.

5. Farmer PE, Nizeye B, Stulac S, Keshavjee S. Structural violence and clinical medicine. PLoS Med. 2006;3(10):e449

6. Gregg J, Saha S. Losing culture on the way to competence: the use and misuse of culture in medical education. Acad Med. 2006;81(6):542–7.

7. Hunt LM. Beyond cultural competence: applying humility to clinical settings [Internet] 2001 [cited 2018 Aug 30]. Available from: https://repository.library.georgetown.edu/handle/10822/950085

8. Jenks AC. From "lists of traits" to "open-mindedness": emerging issues in cultural competence education. Cult Med Psychiatry. 2011;35(2):209–35.

9. Juarez JA, Marvel K, Brezinski KL, Glazner C, Towbin MM, Lawton S. Bridging the gap: a curriculum to teach residents cultural humility. Fam Med. 2006;38(2):97–102.
10. Kleinman A, Benson P. Anthropology in the clinic: the problem of cultural competency and how to fix it. PLoS Med. 2006;3(10):e294.
11. Kumagai AK, Lypson ML. Beyond cultural competence: critical consciousness, social justice, and multicultural education. Acad Med. 2009;84(6):782–7.
12. McGibbon E, Mulaudzi FM, Didham P, Barton S, Sochan A. Toward decolonizing nursing: the colonization of nursing and strategies for increasing the counter-narrative. Nurs Inq. 2014;21(3):179–91.
13. Messac L, Ciccarone D, Draine J, Bourgois P. The Good-enough science-and-politics of anthropological collaboration with evidence-based clinical research: four ethnographic case studies. Soc Sci Med. 2013;99:176–86.
14. Paparella-Pitzel S, Eubanks R, Kaplan SL. Comparison of teaching strategies for cultural humility in physical therapy. J Allied Health. 2016;45(2):139–46.
15. Tervalon M, Murray-García J. Cultural humility versus cultural competence: a critical distinction in defining physician training outcomes in multicultural education. J Health Care Poor Underserved. 1998;9(2):117–25.
16. Wells K, Jones L. "Research" in community-partnered, participatory research. JAMA. 2009;302(3):320–1.
17. Willen SS, Bullon A, Good MJ. Opening up a huge can of worms: reflections on a "cultural sensitivity" course for psychiatry residents. Harv Rev. Psychiatry. 2010;18(4):247–53.

Structural Determinants and Interventions: Public Health Looks Upstream

1. Andermann A. Taking action on the social determinants of health in clinical practice: a framework for health professionals. CMAJ. 2016;188(17–18):E474–83.
2. Beletsky L, Cochrane J, Sawyer AL, Serio-Chapman C, Smelyanskaya M, Han J, et al. Police encounters among needle exchange clients in Baltimore: drug law enforcement as a structural determinant of health. Am J Public Health. 2015;105(9):1872–9.
3. Breilh J. Latin American critical ('social') epidemiology: new settings for an old dream. Int J Epidemiol. 2008;37(4):745–50.
4. Briggs CL, Mantini-Briggs C. Confronting health disparities: Latin American social medicine in Venezuela. Am J Public Health. 2009;99(3):549–55.
5. Chang VW, Lauderdale DS. Fundamental cause theory, technological innovation, and health disparities: the case of cholesterol in the era of statins. J Health Soc Behav. 2009;50(3):245–60.
6. Draine J, McTighe L, Bourgois P. Education, empowerment and community based structural reinforcement: an HIV prevention response to mass incarceration and removal. Int J Law Psychiatry. 2011;34(4):295–302.
7. Fleming MD, Shim JK, Yen IH, Thompson-Lastad A, Rubin S, Van Natta M, et al. Patient engagement at the margins: health care providers' assessments of engagement and the structural determinants of health in the safety-net. Soc Sci Med. 2017;183:11–8.
8. Freudenberg N, Franzosa E, Chisholm J, Libman K. New approaches for moving upstream: how state and local health departments can transform practice to reduce health inequalities. Health Educ Behav. 2015;42(1 Suppl):46S–56S.
9. Geronimus AT. To mitigate, resist, or undo: addressing structural influences on the health of urban populations. Am J Public Health. 2000;90(6):867–72.
10. Gore DM, Kothari AR. Getting to the root of the problem: health promotion strategies to address the social determinants of health. Can J Public Health. 2013;104(1):e52–4.
11. Gottlieb LM, Tirozzi KJ, Manchanda R, Burns AR, Sandel MT. Moving electronic medical records upstream: incorporating social determinants of health. Am J Prev Med. 2015;48(2):215–8.

12. Harvey M, McGladrey M. Explaining the origins and distribution of health and disease: an analysis of epidemiologic theory in core Master of Public Health coursework in the United States. Crit Public Health. 2018;29(1):5–17.
13. Kalofonos IA. "All I eat is ARVs": the paradox of AIDS treatment interventions in Central Mozambique. Med Anthropol Q. 2010;24(3):363–80.
14. Knight KR. addicted.pregnant.poor. Durham: Duke University Press Books; 2015.
15. Laurell AC. What does Latin American social medicine do when it governs? The case of the Mexico City government. Am J Public Health. 2003;93(12):2028–31.
16. Lu T, Zwicker L, Kwena Z, Bukusi E, Mwaura-Muiru E, Dworkin SL. Assessing barriers and facilitators of implementing an integrated HIV prevention and property rights program in Western Kenya. AIDS Educ Prev. 2013;25(2):151–63.
17. National Research Council, Institute of Medicine. U.S. health in international perspective: shorter lives, poorer health [Internet]. Woolf SH, Aron L, editors. Washington, DC: National Academies Press; 2013. Available from: http://www.ncbi.nlm.nih.gov/books/NBK115854/
18. Navarro V. What we mean by social determinants of health. Int J Health Serv. 2009;39(3):423–41.
19. Netherland J, Hansen H. White opioids: pharmaceutical race and the war on drugs that wasn't. BioSocieties. 2017;12(2):217–38.
20. Sommer M, Parker R, editors. Structural approaches in public health. London: Routledge; 2013.
21. Porter D. How did social medicine evolve, and where is it heading? PLoS Med. 2006;3(10):e399.
22. Pronyk PM, Hargreaves JR, Kim JC, Morison LA, Phetla G, Watts C, et al. Effect of a structural intervention for the prevention of intimate-partner violence and HIV in rural South Africa: a cluster randomised trial. Lancet. 2006;368(9551):1973–83.
23. Reich AD, Hansen HB, Link BG. Fundamental interventions: how clinicians can address the fundamental causes of disease. J Bioeth Inq. 2016;13(2):185–92.
24. Sharma M, Pinto AD, Kumagai AK. Teaching the social determinants of health: a path to equity or a road to nowhere? Acad Med. 2018;93(1):25.
25. Wilkinson R, Pickett K. The Spirit level: why greater equality makes societies stronger. Reprint edition. New York: Bloomsbury Press; 2011.
26. Williams DR, Costa MV, Odunlami AO, Mohammed SA. Moving upstream: how interventions that address the social determinants of health can improve health and reduce disparities. J Public Health Manag Pract. 2008;14(Suppl):S8–17.
27. Woolf SH, Johnson RE, Phillips RL, Philipsen M. Giving everyone the health of the educated: an examination of whether social change would save more lives than medical advances. Am J Public Health. 2007;97(4):679–83.

Medical-Legal Partnerships

1. Beck AF, Klein MD, Schaffzin JK, Tallent V, Gillam M, Kahn RS. Identifying and treating a substandard housing cluster using a medical-legal partnership. Pediatrics. 2012;130(5):831–8.
2. Cohen E, Fullerton DF, Retkin R, Weintraub D, Tames P, Brandfield J, et al. Medical-legal partnership: collaborating with lawyers to identify and address health disparities. J Gen Intern Med. 2010;25(Suppl 2):136.
3. Pettignano R, Caley SB, Bliss LR. Medical-legal partnership: impact on patients with sickle cell disease. Pediatrics. 2011;128(6):e1482–8.
4. Regenstein M, Trott J, Williamson A, Theiss J. Addressing social determinants of health through medical-legal partnerships. Health Aff. 2018;37(3):378–85.
5. Sandel M, Hansen M, Kahn R, Lawton E, Paul E, Parker V, et al. Medical-legal partnerships: transforming primary care by addressing the legal needs of vulnerable populations. Health Aff. 2010;29(9):1697–705.
6. Teufel J, Heller SM, Dausey DJ. Medical-legal partnerships as a strategy to improve social causes of stress and disease. Am J Public Health. 2014;104(12):e6.

Advocacy and Activism: Structural Organizing in Action

1. Aksel S, Fein L, Ketterer E, Young E, Backus L. Unintended consequences: abortion training in the years after Roe v Wade. Am J Public Health. 2013;103(3):404.
2. Almond D, Chay KY, Greenstone M. Civil rights, the war on poverty, and black-white convergence in infant mortality in the rural South and Mississippi [Internet]. Rochester: Social Science Research Network; 2006 [cited 2018 Aug 31]. Report No.: ID 961021. Available from: https://papers.ssrn.com/abstract=961021
3. Charles D, Himmelstein K, Keenan W, Barcelo N, White Coats for Black Lives National Working Group. White coats for black lives: medical students responding to racism and police brutality. J Urban Health. 2015;92(6):1007–10.
4. Dobson S, Voyer S, Hubinette M, Regehr G. From the clinic to the community: the activities and abilities of effective health advocates. Acad Med. 2015;90(2):214–20.
5. Drucker E, Anderson K, Haemmig R, Heimer R, Small D, Walley A, et al. Treating addictions: harm reduction in clinical care and prevention. J Bioeth Inq. 2016;13(2):239–49.
6. Fullilove M. Root Shock: How Tearing Up City Neighborhoods Hurts America, and What We Can Do About It. 1st edition. New York: One World/Ballantine; 2004.
7. Fullilove M. Urban Alchemy: restoring joy in America's sorted-out cities. Oakland: New Village Press; 2013.
8. Geiger HJ. The political future of social medicine: reflections on physicians as activists. Acad Med. 2017;92(3):282–4.
9. Keefe RH, Lane SD, Swarts HJ. From the bottom up: tracing the impact of four health-based social movements on health and social policies. J Health Soc Policy. 2006;21(3):55–69.
10. Lefkowitz B. Community Health Centers: a movement and the people who made it happen. None ed. New Brunswick: Rutgers University Press; 2007.
11. Liggett A, Sharma M, Nakamura Y, Villar R, Selwyn P. Results of a voter registration project at 2 family medicine residency clinics in the Bronx, New York. Ann Fam Med. 2014;12(5):466–9.
12. Nelson A. Body and soul: the black panther party and the fight against medical discrimination. 1st ed. Minneapolis/London: University of Minnesota Press; 2013.
13. Saul J. Collective trauma, collective healing: promoting community resilience in the aftermath of disaster. New York: Routledge; 2013.

Film and Television

1. Morales I. Palante, Siempre Palante! [Internet]. A documentary about the Young Lords Party and its community health and education projects among Latinx in the 1970s. [cited 2018 Oct 3]. Available from: http://palante.org/Documentary.htm
2. Scott C. Selling Sickness [Internet]. A documentary about the ways pharmaceutical companies market to consumers. Icarus Films; [cited 2018 Oct 3]. Available from: http://icarusfilms.com/if-sell
3. Out in the Rural: A Health Center in Mississippi [Internet]. A documentary about the first Community Health Center in the 1960, its organizers Dr. H. Jack Geiger and colleagues. Available from: https://www.youtube.com/watch?v=UiunAOZ9iUg
4. Unnatural Causes [Internet]. A miniseries on the social determinants of health. California Newsreel. [cited 2018 Oct 3]. Available from: https://unnaturalcauses.org/about_the_series.php

Websites

1. Structural Competency. [cited 2018 Oct 20]. Available from: https://structuralcompetency.org/
2. Structural Competency Working Group. [cited 2018 Oct 20]. Available from: https://www. structcomp.org
3. Beyond Flexner Alliance: Social Mission in Health Professions Education. [cited 2018 Oct 20]. Available from: http://beyondflexner.org/
4. HealthBegins. [cited 2018 Oct 20]. Available from: https://www.healthbegins.org/

Index

A
Accompaniment, 155
Advocacy
    coalition of, 215
    non-profit organization, 212
    organization, DPA, 211
    organizations, 216
    policy, 211
Affordable Care Act (ACA), 7
Allied health care workers, 191, 201, 203
American myth of exceptionalism, 30
Anthropology, 23

B
Baltimore CONNECT, 21
Behavioral Risk Factor Surveillance System
    (BRFSS), 91
Beloved community, 65
Black Freedom Movement, 28, 29
Bridges Curriculum, 39–43
Buprenorphine, 214

C
Causes of death, student' work, 92
Centers for Disease Control and Prevention
    (CDC), 92
Charity
    care, 193
    cases, 194
    dependent workforce, 194
    of individual supervisors, 197
Child care fund, 200
Child Health-Law Partnership (Child HeLP),
    127
City Life Is Moving Bodies (CLIMB)
    framework, 104
    goal of, 106

Collective development, 31
Collective traumas, 112, 117, 119
Community based participatory research
    (CBPR), 169
Community based partnerships, 204
Community clinic, 20
    Baltimore CONNECT, 21
    East Baltimore Medical Plan, 22
    OB/GYN clinic, 22
    ratings from students, 22
Community engagement, 109, 110
    approach, 144
    definition of, 142
    efforts, 144
    initiative, 145
    and peer collaboration, 139–140
    and resource mapping, 139
Community health, 105
    assessment, 87
    status, 87
Community health assessment (CHA), 89–94
Community health worker (CHW)
    for diabetes care, 170–171
    evidence-based approach, 169
    perspectives of, 170–174
Community medicine fieldwork, 94–95
Community participation, 104
Community resilience, 113
Community-Oriented Primary Care
    (COPC), 88
Concrete totality, 29
Conflict-based knowledge, 27
Criminal justice
    academy of public health and, 182–183
    agencies, 182
    boundaries of, 185
    community health and, 185
    public health and, 182
Cross-sector policy innovations, 187–188

© Springer Nature Switzerland AG 2019
H. Hansen, J. M. Metzl (eds.), *Structural Competency in Mental Health and Medicine*,
https://doi.org/10.1007/978-3-030-10525-9

Printed by Printforce, the Netherlands